Cardiovascular physiology

BY : Ali Ahmed

Left ventricular ejection fraction:
- Left ventricular ejection fraction = (stroke volume / end diastolic LV volume) * 100%
- Stroke volume = end diastolic LV volume - end systolic LV volume

Pulse pressure:
- Pulse pressure = Systolic Pressure - Diastolic Pressure

  Factors which increase pulse pressure
  1) a less compliant aorta (this tends to occur with advancing age)
  2) increased stroke volume

Hypertention

Secondary causes:

- It is thought that between 5-10% of patients diagnosed with hypertension have **primary hyperaldosteronism**, including <u>Conn's syndrome</u>. This makes it the single most common cause of secondary hypertension.
- Renal disease accounts for a large percentage of the other cases of secondary hypertension.
- Conditions which may increase the blood pressure include:
  - glomerulonephritis
  - pyelonephritis
  - adult polycystic kidney disease
  - renal artery stenosis

Endocrine disorders (other than primary hyperaldosteronism) may also result in increased blood pressure:
- phaeochromocytoma
- Cushing's syndrome
- Liddle's syndrome
- congenital adrenal hyperplasia (11-beta hydroxylase deficiency)
- acromegaly

Other causes include:
- NSAIDs

- pregnancy
- coarctation of the aorta
- the combined oral contraceptive pill
- steroids
- MAOI

Isolated systolic hypertension

- Isolated systolic hypertension (ISH) is common in the elderly.
- Affecting around 50% of people older than 70 years old.
- The Systolic Hypertension in the Elderly Program (SHEP) back in 1991 established that treating ISH reduced both strokes and ischaemic heart disease.
- Drugs such as **thiazides** were recommended as first line agents.
- This approach is contradicated by the 2011 NICE guidelines which recommends treating ISH in the same stepwise fashion as standard hypertension.

Hypertension diagnosis:

- NICE published updated guidelines for the management of hypertension in 2011.
- Some of the key changes include:

  ✓ classifying hypertension into stages
  ✓ recommending the use of ambulatory blood pressure monitoring (ABPM) and home blood pressure monitoring (HBPM)

Why were these guidelines needed?

It has long been recognised by doctors that there is a subgroup of patients whose blood pressure climbs 20 mmHg whenever they enter a clinical setting, so called 'white coat hypertension'. If we just rely on clinic readings then such patients may be diagnosed as having hypertension when the vast majority of time there blood pressure is normal.

This has led to the use of both ambulatory blood pressure monitoring (ABPM) and home blood pressure monitoring (HBPM) to confirm the diagnosis of hypertension. These techniques allow a more accurate assessment of a patients' overall blood pressure. Not only does this help prevent overdiagnosis of hypertension - ABPM has been shown to be a more accurate predictor of cardiovascular events than clinic readings.

Blood pressure classification

This becomes relevant later in some of the management decisions that NICE advocate.

Stage	Criteria
Stage 1 hypertension	Clinic BP >= 140/90 mmHg and subsequent ABPM daytime average or HBPM average BP >= 135/85 mmHg
Stage 2 hypertension	Clinic BP >= 160/100 mmHg and subsequent ABPM daytime average or HBPM average BP >= 150/95 mmHg
Severe hypertension	Clinic systolic BP >= 180 mmHg, or clinic diastolic BP >= 110 mmHg

Diagnosing hypertension:

- Firstly, NICE recommend measuring blood pressure in both arms when considering a diagnosis of hypertension.
- If the difference in readings between arms is more than 20 mmHg then the measurements should be repeated.
- If the difference remains > 20 mmHg then subsequent blood pressures should be recorded from the arm with the higher reading.
- It should of course be remember that there are pathological causes of unequal blood pressure readings from the arms, such as **supravalvular aortic stenosis**.
- It is therefore prudent to listen to the heart sounds if a difference exists and further investigation if a very large difference is noted.
- NICE also recommend taking a second reading during the consultation, if the first reading is > 140/90 mmHg. The lower reading of the two should determine further management.
- NICE suggest offering ABPM or HBPM to any patient with a blood pressure >= 140/90 mmHg.
- If however the blood pressure is >= 180/110 mmHg:
  - immediate treatment should be considered
  - if there are signs of papilloedema or retinal haemorrhages NICE recommend same day assessment by a specialist
  - NICE also recommend referral if a phaeochromocytoma is suspected (labile or postural hypotension, headache, palpitations, pallor and diaphoresis)

Ambulatory blood pressure monitoring (ABPM):
- at least 2 measurements per hour during the person's usual waking hours (for example, between 08:00 and 22:00)
- use the average value of at least 14 measurements
- If ABPM is not tolerated or declined HBPM should be offered.

Home blood pressure monitoring (HBPM):
- for each BP recording, two consecutive measurements need to be taken, at least 1 minute apart and with the person seated
- BP should be recorded twice daily, ideally in the morning and evening

- BP should be recorded for at least 4 days, ideally for 7 days

- discard the measurements taken on the first day and use the average value of all the remaining measurements

Interpreting the results
1) **ABPM/HBPM >= 135/85 mmHg (i.e. stage 1 hypertension)**
   - treat if < 80 years of age AND any of the following apply;
     ⇒ target organ damage,
     ⇒ established cardiovascular disease,
     ⇒ renal disease,
     ⇒ diabetes or
     ⇒ a 10-year cardiovascular risk equivalent to 20% or greater
2) **ABPM/HBPM >= 150/95 mmHg (i.e. stage 2 hypertension)**
   - offer drug treatment regardless of age

Hypertension management:
- NICE published updated guidelines for the management of hypertension in 2011.
- Some of the key changes include:
  - classifying hypertension into stages
  - recommending the use of ambulatory blood pressure monitoring (ABPM) and home blood pressure monitoring (HBPM)
  - calcium channel blockers are now considered superior to thiazides
  - bendroflumethiazide is no longer the thiazide of choice

Managing hypertension
1) **Lifestyle advice** should not be forgotten and is frequently tested in exams:
   - A low salt diet is recommended, aiming for less than 6g/day, ideally 3g/day.
   - The average adult in the UK consumes around 8-12g/day of salt.
   - A recent BMJ paper* showed that lowering salt intake can have a significant effect on blood pressure. For example, reducing salt intake by 6g/day can lower systolic blood pressure by 10mmHg
   - caffeine intake should be reduced
   - the other general bits of advice remain: stop smoking, drink less alcohol, eat a balanced diet rich in fruit and vegetables, exercise more, lose weight

2) **ABPM/HBPM >= 135/85 mmHg (i.e. stage 1 hypertension)**
   - treat if < 80 years of age AND any of the following apply; target organ damage, established cardiovascular disease, renal disease, diabetes or a 10-year cardiovascular risk equivalent to 20% or greater

3) **ABPM/HBPM >= 150/95 mmHg (i.e. stage 2 hypertension)**

- offer drug treatment regardless of age

⬇ For patients < 40 years consider specialist referral to exclude secondary causes.

Step 1 treatment:
- patients < 55-years-old: ACE inhibitor (A)
- patients > 55-years-old or of Afro-Caribbean origin: calcium channel blocker

Step 2 treatment:
- ACE inhibitor + calcium channel blocker (A + C)

Step 3 treatment:
- add a thiazide diuretic (D, i.e. A + C + D)
- NICE now advocate using either:
  - ✓ chlorthalidone (12.5-25.0 mg once daily) or
  - ✓ indapamide (1.5 mg modified-release once daily or 2.5 mg once daily) in preference to a conventional thiazide diuretic such as bendroflumethiazide

NICE define a clinic BP >= 140/90 mmHg after step 3 treatment with optimal or best tolerated doses as resistant hypertension. They suggest step 4 treatment or seeking expert advice

Step 4 treatment:
1) consider further diuretic treatment
   - if potassium < 4.5 mmol/l add spironolactone 25mg od
   - if potassium > 4.5 mmol/l add higher-dose thiazide-like diuretic treatment
2) if further diuretic therapy is not tolerated, or is contraindicated or ineffective, consider an alpha- or beta-blocker

Patients who fail to respond to step 4 measures should be referred to a specialist. NICE recommend:
If blood pressure remains uncontrolled with the optimal or maximum tolerated doses of four drugs, seek expert advice if it has not yet been obtained.

Blood pressure targets

	Clinic BP	ABPM / HBPM
Age < 80 years	140/90 mmHg	135/85 mmHg
Age > 80 years	150/90 mmHg	145/85 mmHg

New drugs:

Direct renin inhibitors:
- e.g. Aliskiren (branded as Rasilez)
- by inhibiting renin blocks the conversion of angiotensinogen to angiotensin I
- No trials have looked at mortality data yet. Trials have only investigated fall in blood pressure.
- Initial trials suggest aliskiren reduces blood pressure to a similar extent as angiotensin converting enzyme (ACE) inhibitors or angiotensin-II receptor antagonists
- adverse effects were uncommon in trials although diarrhoea was occasionally seen
- only current role would seem to be in patients who are intolerant of more established antihypertensive drugs

Malignant hypertension

Basics:
- severe hypertension (e.g. >200/130 mmHg)
- occurs in both essential and secondary types
- fibrinoid necrosis of blood vessels, leading to:
  - retinal haemorrhages, exudates, and
  - proteinuria, haematuria due to renal damage (benign nephrosclerosis).
- can lead to cerebral oedema → encephalopathy

Features:
- classically: severe headaches, nausea/vomiting, visual disturbance
- however chest pain and dyspnoea common presenting symptoms
- papilloedema
- severe: encephalopathy (e.g. seizures)

Management:
- reduce diastolic no lower than 100mmHg within 12-24 hrs
- bed rest
- most patients: oral therapy e.g. atenolol
- if severe/encephalopathic: IV sodium nitroprusside/labetol

Hypertension in pregnancy

- NICE published guidance in 2010 on the management of hypertension in pregnancy.
- They also made recommendations on reducing the risk of hypertensive disorders developing in the first place:

- Women who are at high risk of developing pre-eclampsia should take **aspirin 75mg od** from 12 weeks until the birth of the baby. High risk groups include:

    - hypertensive disease during previous pregnancies
    - chronic kidney disease
    - autoimmune disorders such as SLE or antiphospholipid syndrome
    - type 1 or 2 diabetes mellitus

- The classification of hypertension in pregnancy is complicated and varies.
- Remember, in normal pregnancy:
    - blood pressure usually falls in the first trimester (particularly the diastolic), and continues to fall until 20-24 weeks
    - after this time the blood pressure usually increases to pre-pregnancy levels by term
- Hypertension in pregnancy in usually defined as:
    - systolic > 140 mmHg or diastolic > 90 mmHg
    - or an increase above booking readings of > 30 mmHg systolic or > 15 mmHg diastolic

After establishing that the patient is hypertensive they should be categorized into one of the following groups:

Pre-existing hypertension	Pregnancy-induced HTN (PIH; also known as gestational HTN)	Pre-eclampsia
A history of hypertension before pregnancy or an elevated blood pressure > 140/90 mmHg before 20 weeks gestation	Hypertension (as defined above) occurring in the second half of pregnancy (i.e. after 20 weeks)	Pregnancy-induced hypertension in association with proteinuria (> 0.3g / 24 hours)
No proteinuria, no oedema	No proteinuria, no oedema	Oedema may occur but is now less commonly used as a criteria
Occurs in 3-5% of pregnancies and is more common in older women	Occurs in around 5-7% of pregnancies	Occurs in around 5% of pregnancies
	Resolves following birth (typically after one month). Women with PIH are at increased risk of future pre-eclampsia or hypertension later in life	

Pre-eclampsia

- Pre-eclampsia is a condition seen after 20 weeks gestation characterised by:
    - ✓ Pregnancy-induced hypertension in association with
    - ✓ Proteinuria (> 0.3g / 24 hours).
- Oedema used to be third element of the classic triad but is now often not included in the definition as it is not specific
- Pre-eclampsia is important as it predisposes to the following problems:
    - fetal: prematurity, intrauterine growth retardation
    - eclampsia
    - haemorrhage: placental abruption, intra-abdominal, intra-cerebral
    - cardiac failure
    - multi-organ failure

Risk factors:
- \> 40 years old
- nulliparity (or new partner)
- multiple pregnancy
- body mass index > 30 kg/m^2
- diabetes mellitus
- pregnancy interval of more than 10 years
- family history of pre-eclampsia
- previous history of pre-eclampsia
- pre-existing vascular disease such as hypertension or renal disease

Features of severe pre-eclampsia:
- hypertension: typically > 170/110 mmHg and proteinuria as above
- proteinuria: dipstick ++/+++
- headache
- visual disturbance
- papilloedema
- RUQ/epigastric pain
- hyperreflexia
- platelet count < $100 * 10^6$/l, abnormal liver enzymes or HELLP syndrome

Management:
- consensus guidelines recommend treating blood pressure > 160/110 mmHg although many clinicians have a lower threshold
- **Oral labetalol** is now first-line following the 2010 NICE guidelines.
- **Nifedipine** and **hydralazine** may also be used
- Delivery of the baby is the most important and definitive management step. The timing depends on the individual clinical scenario

Eclampsia

- Eclampsia may be defined as the development of seizures in association pre-eclampsia.
- To recap, pre-eclampsia is defined as:
    1) condition seen after 20 weeks gestation
    2) pregnancy-induced hypertension
    3) proteinuria

Magnesium sulphate is used to both prevent seizures in patients with severe pre-eclampsia and treat seizures once they develop. Guidelines on its use suggest the following:

1) should be given once a decision to deliver has been made
2) in eclampsia an IV bolus of 4g over 5-10 minutes should be given followed by an infusion of 1g / hour
3) urine output, reflexes, respiratory rate and oxygen saturations should be monitored during treatment
4) treatment should continue for 24 hours after last seizure or delivery (around 40% of seizures occur post-partum)

Other important aspects of treating severe pre-eclampsia/eclampsia include fluid restriction to avoid the potentially serious consequences of fluid overload

Centrally acting antihypertensives

Examples of centrally acting antihypertensives include:

- methyldopa: used in the management of hypertension during pregnancy
- moxonidine: used in the management of essential hypertension when conventional antihypertensives have failed to control blood pressure
- clonidine: the antihypertensive effect is mediated through stimulating alpha-2 adrenoceptors in the vasomotor centre

Diabetes mellitus: hypertension management

NICE recommend the following blood pressure targets for type 2 diabetics:

- if end-organ damage (e.g. renal disease, retinopathy) ≤ 130/80 mmHg
- otherwise ≤ 140/80 mmHg

- A 2013 Cochrane review casted doubt on the wisdom of lower blood pressure targets for patients with diabetes. It compared patients who had tight blood pressure control (targets ≤ 130/85 mmHg) with more relaxed control (≤ 140-160/90-100 mmHg). Patients who were more tightly controlled had a slightly reduced rate of stroke but otherwise outcomes were not significantly different.
- Because ACE-inhibitors have a renoprotective effect in diabetes they are the first-line antihypertensives recommended for NICE.
- Patients of African or Caribbean family origin should be offered an ACE-inhibitor plus either a thiazide diuretic or calcium channel blocker.
- Further management then reverts to that of non-diabetic patients, as discussed earlier in the module.
- Remember than autonomic neuropathy may result in more postural symptoms in patients taking antihypertensive therapy.
- The routine use of beta-blockers in uncomplicated hypertension should be avoided, particularly when given in combination with thiazides, as they may cause insulin resistance, impair insulin secretion and alter the autonomic response to hypoglycaemia.

Heart Failure

Heart failure: NYHA classification

The New York Heart Association (NYHA) classification is widely used to classify the severity of heart failure:

NYHA Class I:
- no symptoms
- no limitation: ordinary physical exercise does not cause undue fatigue, dyspnoea or palpitations

NYHA Class II:
- mild symptoms
- slight limitation of physical activity: comfortable at rest but ordinary activity results in fatigue, palpitations or dyspnoea

NYHA Class III:
- moderate symptoms
- marked limitation of physical activity: comfortable at rest but less than ordinary activity results in symptoms

NYHA Class IV:
- severe symptoms
- unable to carry out any physical activity without discomfort: symptoms of heart failure are present even at rest with increased discomfort with any physical activity

Heart failure: diagnosis

- NICE issued updated guidelines on diagnosis and management in 2010.
- The choice of investigation is determined by whether the patient has previously had a myocardial infarction or not.

Previous myocardial infarction:
- arrange echocardiogram within 2 weeks

No previous myocardial infarction:
- measure serum natriuretic peptides (BNP)
- if levels are 'high' arrange echocardiogram within 2 weeks
- if levels are 'raised' arrange echocardiogram within 6 weeks

Serum natriuretic peptides

- B-type natriuretic peptide (BNP) is a hormone
- produced mainly by the left ventricular myocardium in response to strain.
- Very high levels are associated with a poor prognosis.

	BNP	NTproBNP
High levels	> 400 pg/ml (116 pmol/litre)	> 2000 pg/ml (236 pmol/litre)
Raised levels	100-400 pg/ml (29-116 pmol/litre)	400-2000 pg/ml (47-236 pmol/litre)
Normal levels	< 100 pg/ml (29 pmol/litre)	< 400 pg/ml (47 pmol/litre)

Factors which alter the BNP level:

Increase BNP levels	Decrease BNP levels
Left ventricular hypertrophy	Obesity
Right ventricular overload	Diuretics
Tachycardia	ACE inhibitors
Ischaemia	Angiotensin 2 receptor blockers
Hypoxaemia (including pulmonary embolism)	Beta-blockers
GFR < 60 ml/min	Aldosterone antagonists
Sepsis	
COPD	
Diabetes	
Age > 70	
Liver cirrhosis	

Heart failure drug management:

A number of drugs have been shown to improve mortality in patients with chronic heart failure:
- ACE inhibitors (SAVE, SOLVD, CONSENSUS)
- spironolactone (RALES)
- beta-blockers (CIBIS)
- hydralazine with nitrates (VHEFT-1)

No long-term reduction in mortality has been demonstrated for loop diuretics such as furosemide.

NICE issued updated guidelines on management in 2010, key points include:
1) first-line treatment for all patients is both an ACE-inhibitor and a beta-blocker
2) second-line treatment is now either an aldosterone antagonist, angiotensin II receptor blocker or a hydralazine in combination with a nitrate
3) if symptoms persist cardiac resynchronisation therapy or digoxin* should be considered
4) diuretics should be given for fluid overload
5) offer annual influenza vaccine
6) offer one-off** pneumococcal vaccine

*digoxin has also not been proven to reduce mortality in patients with heart failure. It may however improve symptoms due to its inotropic properties. Digoxin is strongly indicated if there is coexistent atrial fibrillation

**adults usually require just one dose but those with asplenia, splenic dysfunction or chronic kidney disease need a booster every 5 years

Prescribing in patients with heart failure

The following medications may exacerbate heart failure:
1) thiazolidinediones*: pioglitazone is contraindicated as it causes fluid retention
2) verapamil: negative inotropic effect
3) NSAIDs**/glucocorticoids: should be used with caution as they cause fluid retention
4) class I antiarrhythmics; flecainide (negative inotropic and proarrhythmic effect)

*pioglitazone is now the only thiazolidinedione on the market

**low-dose aspirin is an exception - many patients will have coexistent cardiovascular disease and the benefits of taking aspirin easily outweigh the risks

Angiotensin-converting enzyme inhibitors

- Angiotensin-converting enzyme (ACE) inhibitors are now the established first-line treatment in younger patients with hypertension and are also extensively used to treat heart failure.
- They are known to be less effective in treating hypertensive Afro-Caribbean patients.
- ACE inhibitors are also used to treat diabetic nephropathy and have a role in secondary prevention of ischaemic heart disease.

Mechanism of action:
- inhibit the conversion angiotensin I to angiotensin II

Side-effects:
- Cough: occurs in around 15% of patients and may occur up to a year after starting treatment. Thought to be due to increased bradykinin levels
- angioedema: may occur up to a year after starting treatment
- hyperkalaemia
- first-dose hypotension: more common in patients taking diuretics

Cautions and contraindications:
- pregnancy and breastfeeding - avoid
- renovascular disease - significant renal impairment may occur in patients who have undiagnosed bilateral renal artery stenosis
- aortic stenosis - may result in hypotension
- patients receiving high-dose diuretic therapy (more than 80 mg of furosemide a day) - significantly increases the risk of hypotension
- hereditary of idiopathic angioedema

Monitoring:
- urea and electrolytes should be checked before treatment is initiated and after increasing the dose
- A rise in the creatinine and potassium may be expected after starting ACE inhibitors. Acceptable changes are an increase in serum creatinine, up to 30%* from baseline and an increase in potassium up to 5.5 mmol/l*.

*Renal Association UK; Clinical Knowledge Summaries quote 50% which seems rather high. SIGN advise that the fall in eGFR should be less than 20%. The NICE CKD guidelines suggest that a decrease in eGFR of up to 25% or a rise in creatinine of up to 30% is acceptable

Bendroflumethiazide

- Bendroflumethiazide (bendrofluazide) is a thiazide diuretic which works by inhibiting sodium absorption at the beginning of the distal convoluted tubule (DCT).
- Potassium is lost as a result of more sodium reaching the collecting ducts.
- Bendroflumethiazide has a role in the treatment of mild heart failure although loop diuretics are better for reducing overload.
- The main use of bendroflumethiazide was in the management of hypertension but recent NICE guidelines now recommend other thiazide-like diuretics such as indapamide and chlortalidone.

Common adverse effects:
1) dehydration
2) postural hypotension
3) hyponatraemia; hypokalaemia; hypercalcaemia
4) gout
5) impaired glucose tolerance
6) impotence

Rare adverse effects:
1) thrombocytopaenia
2) agranulocytosis
3) photosensitivity rash
4) pancreatitis

Loop diuretics

- Furosemide and bumetanide are loop diuretics that act by inhibiting the Na-K-Cl cotransporter (NKCC) in the thick ascending limb of the loop of Henle, reducing the absorption of NaCl.
- There are two variants of NKCC; loop diuretics act on NKCC2, which is more prevalent in the kidneys

Indications:
1) heart failure: both acute (usually intravenously) and chronic (usually orally)
2) resistant hypertension, particularly in patients with renal impairment

Adverse effects:
1) hypotension
2) hyponatraemia
3) hypokalaemia
4) hypochloraemic alkalosis
5) ototoxicity
6) hypocalcaemia

7) enal impairment (from dehydration + direct toxic effect)
7) hyperglycaemia (less common than with thiazides)
8) gout

Beta-blocker overdose

Features:
- bradycardia
- hypotension
- heart failure
- syncope

Management:
- if bradycardic then atropine
- in resistant cases glucagon may be used

Haemodialysis is not effective in beta-blocker overdose

Calcium channel blockers

- Calcium channel blockers are primarily used in the management of cardiovascular disease.
- Voltage-gated calcium channels are present in:
    1) myocardial cells,
    2) cells of the conduction system
    3) the vascular smooth muscle cells

The various types of calcium channel blockers have varying effects on these three areas and it is therefore important to differentiate their uses and actions.

Digoxin and digoxin toxicity

- Digoxin is a cardiac glycoside now mainly used for rate control in the management of atrial fibrillation.
- As it has positive inotropic properties it is sometimes used for improving symptoms (but not mortality) in patients with heart failure.

Mechanism of action:
- ✓ decreases conduction through the atrioventricular node which slows the ventricular rate in atrial fibrillation and flutter
- ✓ Increases the force of cardiac muscle contraction due to inhibition of the Na^+/K^+ ATPase pump.
- ✓ Also stimulates vagus nerve

Digoxin toxicity:
- Plasma concentration alone does not determine whether a patient has developed digoxin toxicity.
- The BNF advises that the likelihood of toxicity increases progressively from 1.5 to 3 mcg/l.

Features:
- ➤ generally unwell, lethargy, nausea & vomiting, anorexia, confusion, yellow-green vision

- arrhythmias (e.g. AV block, bradycardia)

Precipitating factors
- classically: hypokalaemia* ,hypomagnesaemia
- hypercalcaemia, hypernatraemia, acidosis
- hypoalbuminaemia
- hypothermia
- hypothyroidism
- increasing age
- renal failure
- myocardial ischaemia
- Drugs:
    - Amiodarone, quinidine,
    - verapamil, diltiazem,
    - spironolactone (competes for secretion in distal convoluted tubule therefore reduce excretion),
    - Ciclosporin.
    - Also drugs which cause hypokalaemia e.g. thiazides and loop diuretics

*hyperkalaemia may also worsen digoxin toxicity, although this is very small print

Management:
- Digibind
- correct arrhythmias
- monitor potassium

ECG: digoxin

ECG features
- down-sloping ST depression ('reverse tick')
- flattened/inverted T waves
- short QT interval
- arrhythmias e.g. AV block, bradycardia

Aspirin

Aspirin works by blocking the action of both cyclooxygenase-1 and 2. Cyclooxygenase is responsible for prostaglandin, prostacyclin and thromboxane synthesis. The blocking of thromboxane A2 formation in platelets reduces the ability of platelets to aggregate which has lead to the widespread use of low-dose aspirin in cardiovascular disease. Until recent guidelines changed all patients with established cardiovascular disease took aspirin if there was no contraindication. Following the 2010 technology appraisal of clopidogrel this is no longer the case*.

Two recent trials (the Aspirin for Asymptomatic Atherosclerosis and the Antithrombotic Trialists Collaboration) have cast doubt on the use of aspirin in primary prevention of cardiovascular disease. Guidelines have not yet changed to reflect this. However the Medicines and Healthcare products Regulatory Agency (MHRA) issued a drug safety update in January 2010 reminding prescribers that aspirin is not licensed for primary prevention.

What do the current guidelines recommend?

- first-line for patients with ischaemic heart disease

Potentiates
- oral hypoglycaemics
- warfarin
- steroids

*NICE now recommend clopidogrel first-line following an ischaemic stroke and for peripheral arterial disease. For TIAs the situation is more complex. Recent Royal College of Physician (RCP) guidelines support the use of clopidogrel in TIAs. However the older NICE guidelines still recommend aspirin + dipyridamole - a position the RCP state is 'illogical'

Dipyridamole

Dipyridamole is an antiplatelet mainly used in combination with aspirin after an ischaemic stroke or transient ischaemic attack.

Mechanism of action
- inhibits phosphodiesterase, elevating platelet cAMP levels which in turn reduce intracellular calcium levels
- other actions include reducing cellular uptake of adenosine and inhibition of thromboxane synthase

IHD

Coronary circulation

Arterial supply of the heart:

- left aortic sinus → left coronary artery (LCA)
- right aortic sinus → right coronary artery (RCA)
- LCA → LAD + circumflex
- RCA → posterior descending
- RCA supplies SA node in 60%; AV node in 90%

Venous drainage of the heart:

- coronary sinus drains into the right atrium

ECG: coronary territories

- The table below shows the correlation between ECG changes and coronary territories:

	ECG changes	Coronary artery
Anteroseptal	V1-V4	Left anterior descending
Inferior	II, III, AVf	Right coronary
Anterolateral	V4-6, I, aVL	Left anterior descending or left circumflex
Lateral	I, aVL +/- V5-6	Left circumflex
Posterior	Tall R waves V1-2	Usually left circumflex; also right coronary

Chest pain:

Assessment of patients with suspected cardiac chest pain

- NICE issued guidelines in 2010 on the 'Assessment and diagnosis of recent onset chest pain or discomfort of suspected cardiac origin'.
- Below is a brief summary of the key points.

Patients presenting with acute chest pain

1) **Immediate management of suspected acute coronary syndrome (ACS):**
   - glyceryl trinitrate
   - aspirin 300mg. NICE do not recommend giving other antiplatelet agents (i.e. Clopidogrel) outside of hospital
   - do not routinely give oxygen; only give if sats < 94%*
   - Perform an ECG as soon as possible but do not delay transfer to hospital.
   - A normal ECG does not exclude ACS

2) **Referral:**
   - current chest pain or chest pain in the last 12 hours with an abnormal ECG: emergency admission
   - chest pain 12-72 hours ago: refer to hospital the same-day for assessment
   - chest pain > 72 hours ago: perform full assessment with ECG and troponin measurement before deciding upon further action

*NICE suggest the following in terms of oxygen therapy:

- do not routinely administer oxygen, but monitor oxygen saturation using pulse oximetry as soon as possible, ideally before hospital admission.
- Only offer supplemental oxygen to:
  - people with oxygen saturation (SpO2) of less than 94% who are not at risk of hypercapnic respiratory failure, aiming for SpO2 of 94-98%
  - people with chronic obstructive pulmonary disease who are at risk of hypercapnic respiratory failure, to achieve a target SpO2 of 88-92% until blood gas analysis is available.

Patients presenting with stable chest pain:

- With all due respect to NICE the guidelines for assessment of patients with stable chest pain are rather complicated.
- They suggest an approach where the risk of a patient having coronary artery disease (CAD) is calculated based on their symptoms (whether they have typical angina, atypical angina or non-anginal chest pain), age, gender and risk factors.
- NICE define anginal pain as the following:

  1. Constricting discomfort in the front of the chest, neck, shoulders, jaw or arms
  2. Precipitated by physical exertion
  3. Relieved by rest or GTN in about 5 minutes

  - patients with all 3 features have typical angina
  - patients with 2 of the above features have atypical angina
  - patients with 1 or none of the above features have non-anginal chest pain

The risk tables are not reproduced here but can be found by clicking on the link.

- If patients have typical anginal symptoms and a risk of CAD is greater than 90% then no further diagnostic testing is required. It should be noted that all men over the age of 70 years who have typical anginal symptoms fall into this category.

- For patients with an estimated risk of 10-90% the following investigations are recommended. Note the absence of the exercise tolerance test:

Estimated likelihood of CAD	Diagnostic testing
61-90%	Coronary angiography
30-60%	Functional imaging, for example: • myocardial perfusion scan with SPECT • stress echocardiography • first-pass contrast-enhanced magnetic resonance (MR) perfusion • MR imaging for stress-induced wall motion abnormalities.
10-29%	CT calcium scoring

Angina pectoris management:

- The management of stable angina comprises lifestyle changes, medication, percutaneous coronary intervention and surgery.
- NICE produced guidelines in 2011 covering **the management of stable angina**

Medication:
- all patients should receive aspirin and a statin in the absence of any contraindication
- sublingual glyceryl trinitrate to abort angina attacks
- NICE recommend using either a beta-blocker or a calicum channel blocker first-line based on 'comorbidities, contraindications and the person's preference'
- If a calcium channel blocker is used as monotherapy a rate-limiting one such as verapamil or diltiazem should be used. If used in combination with a beta-blocker then use a long-acting dihydropyridine calcium-channel blocker (e.g. modified-release nifedipine).
- Remember that beta-blockers should not be prescribed concurrently with verapamil (risk of complete heart block)
    - if there is a poor response to initial treatment then medication should be increased to the maximum tolerated dose (e.g. for atenolol 100mg od)
    - if a patient is still symptomatic after monotherapy with a beta-blocker add a calcium channel blocker and vice versa

- if a patient is on monotherapy and cannot tolerate the addition of a calcium channel blocker or a beta-blocker then consider one of the following drugs: **a long-acting nitrate**, **ivabradine**, **nicorandil** or **ranolazine**
- if a patient is taking both a beta-blocker and a calcium-channel blocker then only add a third drug whilst a patient is awaiting assessment for PCI or CABG

Nitrate tolerance:
- many patients who take nitrates develop tolerance and experience reduced efficacy
- the BNF advises that patients who develop tolerance should take the second dose of isosorbide mononitrate after 8 hours, rather than after 12 hours. This allows blood-nitrate levels to fall for 4 hours and maintains effectiveness
- this effect is not seen in patients who take modified release isosorbide mononitrate

Ivabradine:
- a new class of anti-anginal drug which works by reducing the heart rate
- acts on the I$_f$ ('funny') ion current which is highly expressed in the sinoatrial node, reducing cardiac pacemaker activity
- Adverse effects:
    - ✓ visual effects, particular luminous phenomena, are common.
    - ✓ Bradycardia, due to the mechanism of action, may also be seen
- there is no evidence currently of superiority over existing treatments of stable angina

Acute coronary syndrome:

Prognostic factors:
The 2006 Global Registry of Acute Coronary Events (GRACE) study has been used to derive regression models to predict death in hospital and death after discharge in patients with acute coronary syndrome

Poor prognostic factors:
1) age
2) development (or history) of heart failure
3) peripheral vascular disease
4) reduced systolic blood pressure
5) Killip class*
6) initial serum creatinine concentration
7) elevated initial cardiac markers
8) cardiac arrest on admission
9) ST segment deviation

Killip class = system used to stratify risk post myocardial infarction

Killip class	Features	30 day mortality
I	No clinical signs heart failure	6%
II	Lung crackles; S3	17%
III	Frank pulmonary oedema	38%
IV	Cardiogenic shock	81%

Acute coronary syndrome: Management of NSTEMI

- NICE produced guidelines in 2013 on the Secondary prevention in primary and secondary care for patients following a myocardial infarction management of unstable angina and non-ST elevation myocardial infarction (NSTEMI).
- These superseded the 2010 guidelines which advocated a risk-based approach to management which determined whether drugs such as clopidogrel were given.

A) All patients should receive
1) aspirin 300mg
2) nitrates or morphine to relieve chest pain if required

- Whilst it is common that non-hypoxic patients receive oxygen therapy there is little evidence to support this approach.
- The 2008 British Thoracic Society oxygen therapy guidelines advise not giving oxygen unless the patient is hypoxic.

B) Antithrombin treatment:
- Fondaparinux should be offered to patients who are not at a high risk of bleeding and who are not having angiography within the next 24 hours.
- If angiography is likely within 24 hours or a patient's creatinine is > 265 umol/l **unfractionated heparin should be given**.

C) Clopidogrel 300mg should be given to **all patients and continued for 12 months**.

D) Intravenous glycoprotein IIb/IIIa receptor antagonists
- **Eptifibatide** or **tirofiban**
- It should be given to:
  1) Patients who have an intermediate or higher risk of adverse cardiovascular events (**predicted 6-month mortality above 3.0%**); and
  2) Who are scheduled to undergo angiography within 96 hours of hospital admission

E) Coronary angiography:

- Should be considered within 96 hours of first admission to hospital to patients who have a predicted 6-month mortality above 3.0%.
- It should also be performed as soon as possible in patients who are clinically unstable.

Mechanism of action of drugs commonly used in the management of acute coronary syndrome:

Medication	Mechanism of action
Aspirin	Antiplatelet - inhibits the production of thromboxane A2
Clopidogrel	Antiplatelet - inhibits ADP binding to its platelet receptor
Enoxaparin & Fondaparinux	Activates antithrombin III, which in turn potentiates the inhibition of coagulation factors Xa
Bivalirudin	Reversible direct thrombin inhibitor

Myocardial infarction

Myoglobin rises first following a myocardial infarction

Cardiac enzymes and protein markers

Interpretation of the various cardiac enzymes has now largely been superceded by the introduction of troponin T and I. Questions still however commonly appear in exams.

Key points for the exam
- Myoglobin is the first to rise
- CK-MB is useful to look for reinfarction as it returns to normal after 2-3 days (troponin T remains elevated for up to 10 days)

	Begins to rise	Peak value	Returns to normal
Myoglobin	1-2 hours	6-8 hours	1-2 days
CK-MB	2-6 hours	16-20 hours	2-3 days
CK	4-8 hours	16-24 hours	3-4 days
Trop T	4-6 hours	12-24 hours	7-10 days
AST	12-24 hours	36-48 hours	3-4 days
LDH	24-48 hours	72 hours	8-10 days

Myocardial infarction management:

- A number of studies over the past 10 years have provided an evidence for the management of ST-elevation myocardial infarction (STEMI)
- In the absence of contraindications, all patients should be given:
    - aspirin
    - clopidogrel: the two major studies (CLARITY and COMMIT) both confirmed benefit but used different loading doses (300mg and 75mg respectively)
    - low molecular weight heparin

NICE suggest the following in terms of oxygen therapy:
- do not routinely administer oxygen, but monitor oxygen saturation using pulse oximetry as soon as possible, ideally before hospital admission.
- Only offer supplemental oxygen to:
    - people with oxygen saturation (SpO2) of less than 94% who are not at risk of hypercapnic respiratory failure, aiming for SpO2 of 94-98%
    - people with chronic obstructive pulmonary disease who are at risk of hypercapnic respiratory failure, to achieve a target SpO2 of 88-92% until blood gas analysis is available.

- Primary percutaneous coronary intervention (PCI) has emerged as the gold-standard treatment for STEMI but is not available in all centres.
- Thrombolysis should be performed in patients without access to primary PCI
- With regards to thrombolysis:

    - tissue plasminogen activator (tPA) has been shown to offer clear mortality benefits over streptokinase
    - tenecteplase is easier to administer and has been shown to have non-inferior efficacy to alteplase with a similar adverse effect profile
    - An ECG should be performed 90 minutes following thrombolysis to assess whether there has been a greater than 50% resolution in the ST elevation

- if there has not been adequate resolution then rescue PCI is superior to repeat thrombolysis

- for patients successfully treated with thrombolysis PCI has been shown to be beneficial. The optimal timing of this is still under investigation

Glycaemic control in patients with diabetes mellitus:
- in 2011 NICE issued guidance on the management of hyperglycaemia in acute coronary syndromes
- it recommends using a dose-adjusted insulin infusion with regular monitoring of blood glucose levels to glucose below 11.0 mmol/l
- intensive insulin therapy (an intravenous infusion of insulin and glucose with or without potassium, sometimes referred to as 'DIGAMI') regimes are not recommended routinely

Percutaneous coronary intervention (PCI)

- PCI is a technique used to restore myocardial perfusion in patients with ischaemic heart disease, both in patients with stable angina and acute coronary syndromes.
- Stents are implanted in around 95% of patients - it is now rare for just balloon angioplasty to be performed
- Following stent insertion migration and proliferation of smooth muscle cells and fibroblasts occur to the treated segment. The stent struts eventually become covered by endothelium. Until this happens there is an increased risk of platelet aggregation leading to thrombosis.

Two main complications may occur:

1) Stent thrombosis:
- Due to platelet aggregation as above.
- Occurs in 1-2% of patients.
- Most commonly in the first month.
- Usually presents with acute myocardial infarction

2) Restenosis:
- Due to excessive tissue proliferation around stent.
- Occurs in around 5-20% of patients.
- Most commonly in the first 3-6 months.
- Usually presents with the recurrence of angina symptoms.
- Risk factors include diabetes, renal impairment and stents in venous bypass grafts

Types of stent:
- bare-metal stent (BMS)
- Drug-eluting stents (DES):
  - ✓ Stent coated with paclitaxel or rapamycin which inhibit local tissue growth.
  - ✓ This reduces restenosis rates
  - ✓ The stent thrombosis rates are increased as the process of stent endothelisation is slowed

- Following insertion the most important factor in preventing stent thrombosis is antiplatelet therapy.
- Aspirin should be continued indefinitely.
- The length of clopidogrel treatment depends on the type of stent, reason for insertion and consultant preference

Thrombolysis:

- Thrombolytic drugs activate plasminogen to form plasmin.
- This in turn degrades fibrin and help breaks up thrombi.
- They in primarily used in patients who present with a ST elevation myocardial infarction.
- Other indications include acute ischaemic stroke and pulmonary embolism, although strict inclusion criteria apply.

Examples:
- alteplase
- tenecteplase
- streptokinase

Contraindications to thrombolysis:
- active internal bleeding
- recent haemorrhage, trauma or surgery (including dental extraction)
- coagulation and bleeding disorders
- intracranial neoplasm
- stroke < 3 months
- aortic dissection
- recent head injury
- pregnancy
- severe hypertension

Side-effects:
- haemorrhage
- hypotension - more common with streptokinase
- allergic reactions may occur with streptokinase

Myocardial infarction: secondary prevention

- NICE produced guidelines on the management of patients following a myocardial infarction (MI) in 2013.
- Some key points are listed below

1) **All patients should be offered the following drugs:**
   - dual antiplatelet therapy (aspirin plus a second antiplatelet agent)
   - ACE inhibitor
   - beta-blocker
   - statin

2) **Some selected lifestyle points:**

Diet: advise a Mediterranean style diet, switch butter and cheese for plant oil based products. Do not recommend omega-3 supplements or eating oily fish

Exercise: advise 20-30 mins a day until patients are 'slightly breathless'

Sexual activity
- ✓ may resume 4 weeks after an uncomplicated MI.
- ✓ Reassure patients that sex does not increase their likelihood of a further MI.
- ✓ PDE5 inhibitors (e.g, sildenafil) may be used 6 months after a MI.
- ✓ They should however be avoided in patient prescribed either nitrates or nicorandil

Clopidogrel:
since clopidogrel came off patent it is now much more widely used post-MI

STEMI:
- ✓ The European Society of Cardiology recommend dual antiplatelets for 12 months.
- ✓ In the UK this means aspirin + clopidogrel

Non-ST segment elevation myocardial infarction (NSTEMI):
- ✓ following the NICE2013 Secondary prevention in primary and secondary care for patients following a myocardial infarction guidelines clopidogrel should be given for the first 12 months

Aldosterone antagonists:
- patients who have had an acute MI and who have symptoms and/or signs of heart failure and left ventricular systolic dysfunction, treatment with an aldosterone antagonist licensed for post-MI treatment (e.g. eplerenone) should be initiated within 3-14 days of the MI, preferably after ACE inhibitor therapy

Clopidogrel:
- Clopidogrel is an antiplatelet agent used in the management of cardiovascular disease.

- It was previously used when aspirin was not tolerated or contraindicated but there are now a number of conditions for which clopidogrel is used in addition to aspirin, for example in patients with an acute coronary syndrome.
- Following the 2010 NICE technology appraisal clopidogrel is also now first-line in patients following an ischaemic stroke and in patients with peripheral arterial disease.
- Clopidogrel belongs to a class of drugs known as thienopyridines which have a similar mechanism of action.
- Other examples include:
    - ✓ prasugrel
    - ✓ ticagrelor
    - ✓ ticlopidine

Mechanism:
- antagonist of the $P2Y_{12}$ adenosine diphosphate (ADP) receptor, inhibiting the activation of platelets

Interactions:
- concurrent use of proton pump inhibitors (PPIs) may make clopidogrel less effective (MHRA July 2009)
- This advice was updated by the MHRA in April 2010, evidence seems inconsistent but omeprazole and esomeprazole still cause for concern. Other PPIs such as lansoprazole should be OK - please see the link for more details

Myocardial infarction complications:

Patients are at risk of a number of immediate, early and late complications following a myocardial infarction (MI).

Cardiac arrest:
- This most commonly occurs due to patients developing ventricular fibrillation and is the most common cause of death following a MI.
- Patients are managed as per the ALS protocol with defibrillation.

Cardiogenic shock:
- If a large part of the ventricular myocardium is damaged in the infarction the ejection fraction of the heart may decrease to the point that the patient develops cardiogenic shock.
- This is difficult to treat.
- Other causes of cardiogenic shock include the 'mechanical' complications such as left ventricular free wall rupture as listed below.
- Patients may require inotropic support and/or an intra-aortic balloon pump.

Chronic heart failure:

- As described above, if the patient survives the acute phase their ventricular myocardium may be dysfunctional resulting in chronic heart failure.
- Loop diuretics such as furosemide will decrease fluid overload.
- Both ACE-inhibitors and beta-blockers have been shown to improve the long-term prognosis of patients with chronic heart failure.

Tachyarrhythmias:
- Ventricular fibrillation, as mentioned above, is the most common cause of death following a MI.
- Other common arrhythmias including ventricular tachycardia.

Bradyarrhythmias:
- Atrioventricular block is more common following inferior myocardial infarctions.

Pericarditis:
- Pericarditis in the first 48 hours following a transmural MI is common (c. 10% of patients).
- The pain is typical for pericarditis (worse on lying flat etc),
- a pericardial rub may be heard and
- a pericardial effusion may be demonstrated with an echocardiogram.

Dressler's syndrome:
- Tends to occur around 2-6 weeks following a MI.
- The underlying pathophysiology is thought to be an autoimmune reaction against antigenic proteins formed as the myocardium recovers.
- It is characterised by a combination of fever, pleuritic pain, pericardial effusion and a raised ESR.
- It is treated with NSAIDs.

Left ventricular aneurysm:
- The ischaemic damage sustained may weaken the myocardium resulting in aneurysm formation.
- This is typically associated with persistent ST elevation and left ventricular failure.
- Thrombus may form within the aneurysm increasing the risk of stroke.
- Patients are therefore anticoagulated.

Left ventricular free wall rupture:
- This is seen in around 3% of MIs and occurs around 1-2 weeks afterwards.
- Patients present with acute heart failure secondary to cardiac tamponade (raised JVP, pulsus paradoxus, diminished heart sounds).
- Urgent pericardiocentesis and thoracotomy are required.

Ventricular septal defect:
- Rupture of the interventricular septum usually occurs in the first week and is seen in around 1-2% of patients.

- Features: acute heart failure associated with a pan-systolic murmur.
- An echocardiogram is diagnostic and will exclude acute mitral regurgitation which presents in a similar fashion.
- Urgent surgical correction is needed.

Acute mitral regurgitation:
- More common with infero-posterior infarction and may be due to ischaemia or rupture of the papillary muscle.
- An early-to-mid systolic murmur is typically heard.
- Patients are treated with vasodilator therapy but often require emergency surgical repair.

Exercise tolerance tests: (ETT; also exercise ECG)

Indications: (ETT has a sensitivity of around 80% and a specificity of 70% for ischaemic heart disease)
- assessing patients with suspected angina - however the 2010 NICE Chest pain of recent onset guidelines do not support the use of ETTs for all patients
- risk stratifying patients following a myocardial infarction
- assessing exercise tolerance
- risk stratifying patients with hypertrophic cardiomyopathy

Heart rate:
- maximum predicted heart rate = 220 - patient's age
- the target heart rate is at least 85% of maximum predicted to allow reasonable interpretation of a test as low-risk or negative

Contraindications:
- myocardial infarction less than 7 days ago
- unstable angina
- uncontrolled hypertension (systolic BP > 180 mmHg) or hypotension (systolic BP ≤ 90 mmHg)
- aortic stenosis
- left bundle branch block: this would make the ECG very difficult to interpret

Stop if:
- exhaustion / patient request
- 'severe', 'limiting' chest pain
- ≥ 2mm ST elevation. Stop if rapid ST elevation and pain
- ≥ 3mm ST depression
- systolic blood pressure > 230 mmHg
- systolic blood pressure falling > 20 mmHg
- attainment of maximum predicted heart rate
- heart rate falling > 20% of starting rate

- arrhythmia develops

Exercise: physiological changes

Blood pressure
- systolic increases, diastolic decreases
- leads to increased pulse pressure
- in healthy young people the increase in MABP is only slight

Cardiac output:
- increase in cardiac output may be 3-5 fold
- results from venous constriction, vasodilation and increased myocardial contractibility, as well as from the maintenance of right atrial pressure by an increase in venous return
- heart rate up to 3-fold increase
- stroke volume up to 1.5-fold increase

Hyperlipidaemia Management:

- In 2014 NICE updated their guidelines on lipid modification.
- This proved highly controversial as it meant that we should be recommending statins to a significant proportion of the population over the age of 60 years.
- Anyway, the key points of the new guidelines are summarised below.

Primary prevention:

Who and how to assess risk

- A systematic strategy should be used to identify people aged over 40 years who are likely to be at high risk of cardiovascular disease (CVD), defined as a 10-year risk of **10%** or greater.
- NICE recommend we use the **QRISK2** CVD risk assessment tool for patients aged <= 84 years. Patients >= 85 years are at high risk of CVD due to their age.

- QRISK2 should not be used in the following situations as there are more specific guidelines for these patient groups:
  - type 1 diabetics
  - patients with an estimated glomerular filtration rate (eGFR) less than 60 ml/min and/or albuminuria
  - patients with a history of familial hyperlipidaemia

NICE suggest QRISK2 may underestimate CVD risk in the following population groups:
  - people treated for HIV
  - people with serious mental health problems
  - people taking medicines that can cause dyslipidaemia such as antipsychotics, corticosteroids or immunosuppressant drugs
  - people with autoimmune disorders/systemic inflammatory disorders such as SLE

Measuring lipid levels
- When measuring lipids:

- ✓ Both the total cholesterol and HDL should be checking to provide the most accurate risk of CVD.
- ✓ A full lipid profile should also be checked (i.e. including triglycerides) before starting a statin.
- ✓ The samples do not need to be fasting.
- In the vast majority of patient the cholesterol measurements will be fed into the QRISK2 tool.
- If however the patient's cholesterol is very high we should consider familial hyperlipidaemia.
- NICE recommend the following that we should **consider the possibility of familial hypercholesterolaemia** and investigate further **if:**
  1) **The total cholesterol concentration is > 7.5 mmol/l** and there is a family history of premature coronary heart disease.
  2) **Total cholesterol > 9.0 mmol/l or a non-HDL cholesterol (i.e. LDL) of > 7.5 mmol/l** even in the absence of a first-degree family history of premature coronary heart disease.

Interpreting the QRISK2 result

- Probably the headline changes in the 2014 guidelines were the new, **lower cut-off of 10-year CVD risk cut-off of 10%**.
- **NICE now recommend we offer a statin** to people with **a QRISK2 10-year risk of >= 10%**
- Lifestyle factors are of course important and NICE recommend that we give patients the option of having their CVD risk reassessed after a period of time before starting a statin.
- **Atorvastatin 20mg** should be offered **first-line**.

Special situations:

1) **Type 1 diabetes mellitus:**
   - NICE recommend that we 'consider statin treatment for the primary prevention of CVD in all adults with type 1 diabetes'
   - atorvastatin 20 mg should be offered if type 1 diabetics who are:
     → Older than 40 years, or
     → have had diabetes for more than 10 years or
     → have established nephropathy or
     → have other CVD risk factors

2) **Chronic kidney disease (CKD):**
   - atorvastatin 20mg should be offered to patients with CKD
   - Increase the dose if a greater than 40% reduction in non-HDL cholesterol is not achieved and the eGFR > 30 ml/min.
   - If the eGFR is < 30 ml/min a renal specialist should be consulted before increasing the dose

Secondary prevention
- All patients with CVD should be taking a statin in the absence of any contraindication.
- Atorvastatin 80mg should be offered first-line.

Follow-up of people started on statins:
- NICE recommend we follow-up patients at 3 months
- repeat a full lipid profile
- if the non-HDL cholesterol has not fallen by at least 40% concordance and lifestyle changes should be discussed with the patient
- NICE recommend we consider increasing the dose of atorvastatin up to 80mg

Lifestyle modifications
These are in many ways predictable but NICE make a number of specific points:

1) Cardioprotective diet
   - total fat intake should be <= 30% of total energy intake
   - saturated fats should be <= 7% of total energy intake
   - intake of dietary cholesterol should be < 300 mg/day
   - saturated fats should be replaced by monounsaturated and polyunsaturated fats where possible
   - replace saturated and monounsaturated fat intake with olive oil, rapeseed oil or spreads based on these oils
   - choose wholegrain varieties of starchy food
   - reduce their intake of sugar and food products containing refined sugars including fructose
   - eat at least 5 portions of fruit and vegetables per day
   - eat at least 2 portions of fish per week, including a portion of oily fish
   - eat at least 4 to 5 portions of unsalted nuts, seeds and legumes per week

2) Physical activity:
   - each week aim for at least 150 minutes of moderate intensity aerobic activity or 75 minutes of vigorous intensity aerobic activity or a mix of moderate and vigorous aerobic activity
   - do muscle strengthening activities on 2 or more days a week that work all major muscle groups (legs, hips, back, abdomen, chest, shoulders and arms) in line with national guidance for the general population

3) Weight management:
   - no specific advice is given, overweight patients should be managed in keeping with relevant NICE guidance

4) Alcohol intake:
   - again no specific advice, other than the general recommendation that males drink no more than 3-4 units/day and females no more than 2-3 units/day

5) Smoking cessation:
   - smokers should be encouraged to quit

Familial Hypercholesterolaemia

- FH is an autosomal dominant condition that is thought to affect around 1 in 500 people.
- It results in high levels of LDL-cholesterol which, if untreated, may cause early cardiovascular disease (CVD).
- FH is caused by mutations in the gene which encodes the LDL-receptor protein.

Clinical diagnosis is now based on the Simon Broome criteria

The Simon Broome criteria:

1) in adults total cholesterol (TC) > 7.5 mmol/l and LDL-C > 4.9 mmol/l or
   Children TC > 6.7 mmol/l and LDL-C > 4.0 mmol/l;

plus:

1) **For definite FH**:
   - tendon xanthoma in patients or 1st or 2nd degree relatives or
   - DNA-based evidence of FH

2) **For possible FH**: family history of myocardial infarction:
   - below age 50 years in 2nd degree relative,
   - below age 60 in 1st degree relative, or
   - a family history of raised cholesterol levels

Management

- the use of CVD risk estimation using standard tables is not appropriate in FH as they do not accurately reflect the risk of CVD
- referral to a specialist lipid clinic is usually required
- **the maximum dose of potent statins are usually required**
- **First-degree relatives have a 50% chance** of having the disorder and should therefore be offered screening. This includes children who should be screened by the age of 10 years if there is one affected parent
- **statins should be discontinued in women 3 months before conception** due to the risk of congenital defects

Remnant Hyperlipidaemia:

Overview:

- rare cause of mixed hyperlipidaemia (raised cholesterol and triglyceride levels)
- also known as Fredrickson type III hyperlipidaemia, broad-beta disease and dysbetalipoproteinaemia
- associated with apo-e2 homozygosity
- high incidence of ischaemic heart disease and peripheral vascular disease
- thought to be caused by impaired removal of intermediate density lipoprotein from the circulation by the liver

Features:

- yellow palmar creases
- palmer xanthomas
- tuberous xanthomas

Management:
- fibrates are first line treatment

Hyperlipidaemia xanthomata:
Characteristic xanthomata seen in hyperlipidaemia:

1) **Palmar xanthoma**
   - remnant hyperlipidaemia
   - may less commonly be seen in familial hypercholesterolaemia

2) **Eruptive xanthoma**
   - are due to high triglyceride levels and
   - present as multiple red/yellow vesicles on the extensor surfaces (e.g. elbows, knees)

   Causes of eruptive xanthoma:
   - ✓ familial hypertriglyceridaemia
   - ✓ lipoprotein lipase deficiency

3) **Tendon xanthoma, tuberous xanthoma, xanthelasma:**
   - familial hypercholesterolaemia
   - remnant hyperlipidaemia
   - Xanthelasma are also seen without lipid abnormalities

   Management of xanthelasma, options include:
   - surgical excision
   - topical trichloroacetic acid
   - laser therapy
   - electrodesiccation

Current treatment targets advocate desirable HDL-C levels > 1 mmol/l and plasma TG < 1.7 mmol/l in subjects at risk of CVD.

Hyperlipidaemia: secondary causes:
Causes of predominantly hypertriglyceridaemia:
- diabetes mellitus (types 1 and 2)
- obesity
- alcohol
- chronic renal failure
- drugs: thiazides, non-selective beta-blockers, unopposed oestrogen
- liver disease

Causes of predominantly hypercholesterolaemia
- nephrotic syndrome
- cholestasis
- hypothyroidism

Statins

Statins inhibit the action of HMG-CoA reductase, the rate-limiting enzyme in hepatic cholesterol synthesis

Adverse effects:
1) Myopathy:
    - Includes myalgia, myositis, rhabdomyolysis and asymptomatic raised creatine kinase.
    - Risks factors for myopathy include advanced age, female sex, low body mass index and presence of multisystem disease such as diabetes mellitus.
    - Myopathy is more common in lipophilic statins (simvastatin, atorvastatin) than relatively hydrophilic statins (rosuvastatin, pravastatin, fluvastatin)

2) Liver impairment:
    - The 2014 NICE guidelines recommend checking LFTs at baseline, 3 months and 12 months.
    - Treatment should be discontinued if serum transaminase concentrations rise to and persist at 3 times the upper limit of the reference range

3) There is some evidence that statins may increase the risk of intracerebral haemorrhage in patients who've previously had a stroke. This effect is not seen in primary prevention. For this reason the Royal College of Physicians recommend **avoiding statins in patients with a history of intracerebral haemorrhage**

Who should receive a statin?
1) all people with established cardiovascular disease (stroke, TIA, ischaemic heart disease, peripheral arterial disease)
2) following the 2014 update, NICE recommend anyone with a 10-year cardiovascular risk >= 10%
3) patients with type 2 diabetes mellitus should now be assessed using QRISK2 like other patients are, to determine whether they should be started on statins

Statins should be taken at night as this is when the majority of cholesterol synthesis takes place. This is especially true for simvastatin which has a shorter half-life than other statins

Current guidelines for lipid lowering*

	Total cholesterol (mmol/l)	LDL cholesterol
Joint British Societies	≤ 4.0	≤ 2.0
National Service Framework for CHD	≤ 5.0	≤ 3.0
SIGN 2007	≤ 5.0	≤ 3.0

Nicotinic acid

- Nicotinic acid is used in the treatment of patients with hyperlipidaemia, although its use is limited by side-effects.
- As well as lowering cholesterol and triglyceride concentrations it also raises HDL levels

Adverse effects:
1) flushing
2) impaired glucose tolerance
3) myositis

Myocarditis:

Causes:
- viral: coxsackie; HIV
- bacteria: diphtheria; clostridia
- spirochaetes: Lyme disease
- protozoa: Chagas' disease; toxoplasmosis
- autoimmune
- drugs: doxorubicin

Presentation:
- usually young patient with acute history
- chest pain; SOB;

Cardiac tamponade

Features:
- dyspnoea
- raised JVP, with an absent Y descent - this is due to the limited right ventricular filling
- tachycardia
- hypotension
- muffled heart sounds
- pulsus paradoxus
- Kussmaul's sign (much debate about this)

- ECG: electrical alternans

The key differences between constrictive pericarditis and cardiac tamponade are summarised in the table below:

	Cardiac tamponade	Constrictive pericarditis
JVP	Absent Y descent	X + Y present
Pulsus paradoxus	Present	Absent
Kussmaul's sign	Rare	Present
Characteristic features		Pericardial calcification on CXR

Kussmaul's sign Paradoxical rise in JVP during inspiration

A commonly used mnemonic to remember the absent Y descent in cardiac tamponade is TAMponade = TAMpaX

Cardiomyopathy

Restrictive cardiomyopathy:
Features:
- similar to constrictive Pericarditis
- Features suggesting restrictive cardiomyopathy rather than constrictive pericarditis
    - prominent apical pulse
    - absence of pericardial calcification on CXR
    - heart may be enlarged
    - ECG abnormalities e.g. bundle branch block; Q waves

Causes:
- amyloidosis (e.g. secondary to myeloma) - most common cause in UK
- haemochromatosis
- Loffler's syndrome
- sarcoidosis
- scleroderma

Dilated cardiomyopathy
- dilated heart leading to systolic (+/- diastolic) dysfunction
- all 4 chambers affected but LV more so than RV
- features include arrhythmias; emboli; mitral regurgitation

- absence of congenital, valvular or ischaemic heart disease

Causes often considered separate entities:
- alcohol: may improve with thiamine
- postpartum
- hypertension

Other causes:
- inherited (see below)
- infections e.g. Coxsackie B, HIV, diphtheria, parasitic
- endocrine e.g. Hyperthyroidism
- infiltrative* e.g. Haemochromatosis, sarcoidosis
- neuromuscular e.g. Duchenne muscular dystrophy
- nutritional e.g. Kwashiorkor, pellagra, thiamine/selenium deficiency
- drugs e.g. Doxorubicin

*these causes may also lead to restrictive cardiomyopathy

Inherited dilated cardiomyopathy:
- around a third of patients with DCM are thought to have a genetic predisposition
- a large number of heterogeneous defects have been identified
- the majority of defects are inherited in an autosomal dominant fashion although other patterns of inheritance are seen

Hypertrophic obstructive cardiomyopathy: (HOCM)
- Is an autosomal dominant disorder of muscle tissue
- Caused by defects in the genes encoding contractile proteins.
- The most common defects involve a mutation in the gene encoding:
  - β-myosin heavy chain protein or
  - myosin binding protein C.
  - alpha-tropomyosin and troponin T have been identified.
- The estimated prevalence is 1 in 500.
- It is an important cause of sudden death in apparently healthy individuals.

Features:
- often asymptomatic
- Septal hypertrophy causes left ventricular outflow obstruction
- dyspnoea, angina, syncope
- sudden death (most commonly due to ventricular arrhythmias), arrhythmias, heart failure
- jerky pulse, large 'a' waves, double apex beat
- ejection systolic murmur: increases with Valsalva manoeuvre and decreases on squatting

Associations:
- Friedreich's ataxia

- Wolff-Parkinson White

Echo - mnemonic - MR SAM ASH

- mitral regurgitation (MR)
- systolic anterior motion (SAM) of the anterior mitral valve leaflet
- asymmetric hypertrophy (ASH)

ECG:
- left ventricular hypertrophy
- progressive T wave inversion
- deep Q waves
- atrial fibrillation may occasionally be seen

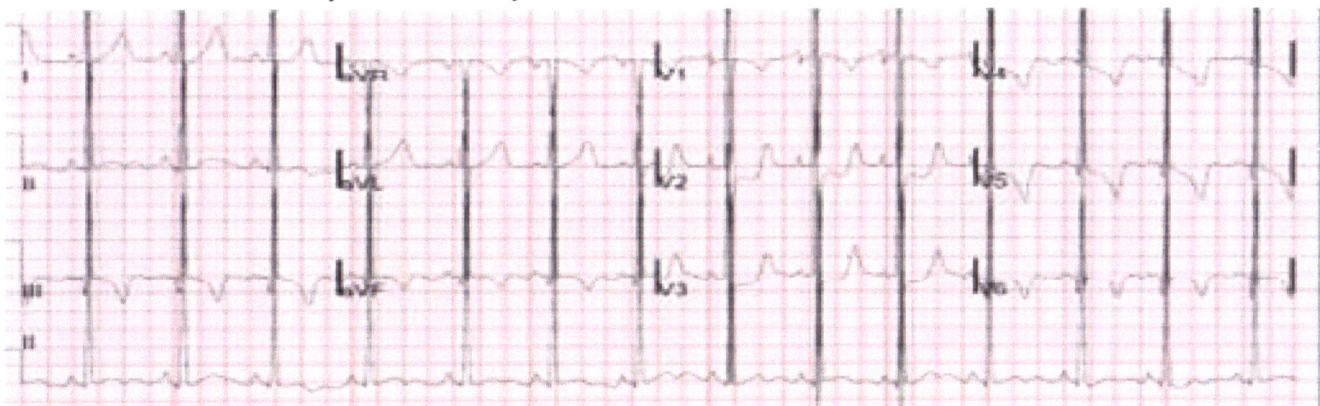

ECG showing typical changes of HOCM including LVH and T wave inversion

Management:
- **A**miodarone
- **B**eta-blockers or verapamil for symptoms
- **C**ardioverter defibrillator
- **D**ual chamber pacemaker
- **E**ndocarditis prophylaxis*

Drugs to avoid:
- nitrates
- ACE-inhibitors
- inotropes

*although see the 2008 NICE guidelines on infective endocarditis prophylaxis

Poor prognostic factors
- syncope
- family history of sudden death
- young age at presentation
- non-sustained ventricular tachycardia on 24 or 48-hour Holter monitoring

- abnormal blood pressure changes on exercise
- An increased septal wall thickness is also associated with a poor prognosis.

Brugada syndrome

- Brugada syndrome is a form of inherited cardiovascular disease with may present with sudden cardiac death.
- It is inherited in an autosomal dominant fashion and
- Has an estimated prevalence of 1:5,000-10,000.
- Brugada syndrome is more common in Asians.

Pathophysiology:
- a large number of variants exist
- around 20-40% of cases are caused by a mutation in the SCN5A gene which encodes the myocardial sodium ion channel protein

ECG changes:
- convex ST segment elevation > 2mm in > 1 of V1-V3 followed by a negative T wave
- partial right bundle branch block
- changes may be more apparent following flecainide

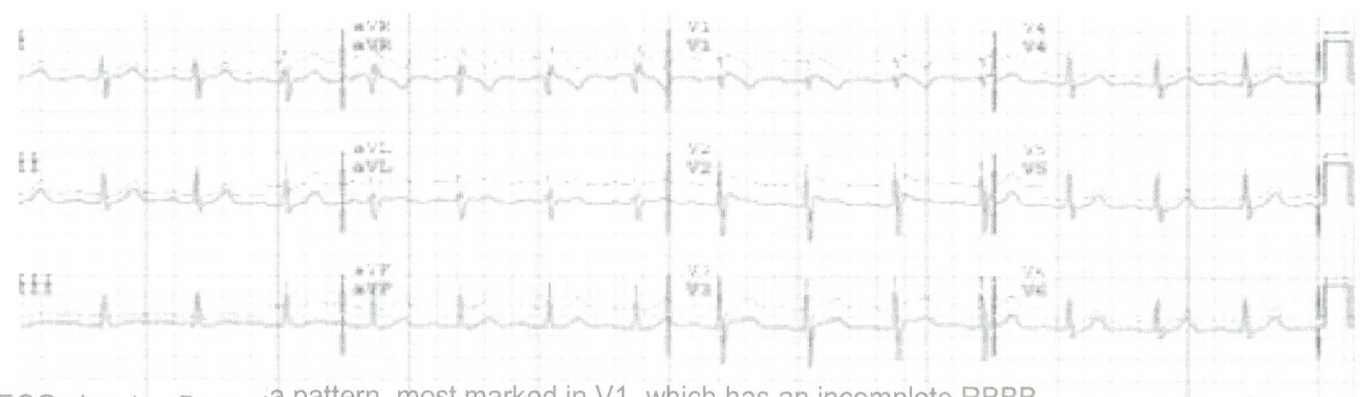

ECG showing Brugada pattern, most marked in V1, which has an incomplete RBBB, a downsloping ST segment and an inverted T wave

Management:
- implantable cardioverter-defibrillator

Arrhythmogenic right ventricular cardiomyopathy (ARVC)

- also known as arrhythmogenic right ventricular dysplasia (ARVD)
- A form of inherited cardiovascular disease which may present with syncope or sudden cardiac death.
- It is generally regarded as the second most common cause of sudden cardiac death in the young after hypertrophic cardiomyopathy.

Pathophysiology:
- inherited in an autosomal dominant pattern with variable expression
- the right ventricular myocardium is replaced by fibrofatty tissue

Presentation:
- palpitations
- syncope
- sudden cardiac death

Investigation:
- ECG abnormalities:
  - In V1-3, typically T wave inversion.
  - An epsilon wave is found in about 50% of those with ARV - this is best described as a terminal notch in the QRS complex
- echo changes are often subtle in the early stages but may show an enlarged, hypokinetic right ventricle with a thin free wall
- magnetic resonance imaging is useful to show fibrofatty tissue

Management:
- drugs: sotalol is the most widely used antiarrhythmic
- catheter ablation to prevent ventricular tachycardia
- implantable cardioverter-defibrillator

Naxos disease:
- an autosomal recessive variant of ARVC
- a triad of ARVC, palmoplantar keratosis, and woolly hair

Catecholaminergic polymorphic ventricular tachycardia (CPVT)

- A form of inherited cardiac disease associated with sudden cardiac death.
- It is inherited in an autosomal dominant fashion and
- Has a prevalence of around 1:10,000.

Pathophysiology:
- the most common cause is a defect in the ryanodine receptor (RYR2) which is found in the myocardial sarcoplasmic reticulum

Features:
- exercise or emotion induced polymorphic ventricular tachycardia resulting in syncope
- sudden cardiac death
- symptoms generally develop before the age of 20 years

Management:
- beta-blockers
- implantable cardioverter-defibrillator

Arrhythmia

ECG: normal variants

The following ECG changes are considered normal variants in an athlete:
- sinus bradycardia
- junctional rhythm
- first degree heart block
- Wenckebach phenomenon

ECG: PR interval

Causes of a **prolonged PR interval**:
- idiopathic
- ischaemic heart disease
- digoxin toxicity
- hypokalaemia*
- rheumatic fever
- aortic root pathology e.g. abscess secondary to endocarditis
- Lyme disease
- sarcoidosis
- myotonic dystrophy
- A prolonged PR interval may also be seen in athletes

A **short PR interval** is seen in Wolff-Parkinson-White syndrome

*hyperkalaemia can rarely cause a prolonged PR interval, but this is a much less common association than hypokalaemia

ECG: ST depression

Causes of ST depression
- secondary to abnormal QRS (LVH, LBBB, RBBB)
- ischaemia
- digoxin
- hypokalaemia
- syndrome X

ECG: ST elevation

Causes of ST elevation:
- myocardial infarction
- pericarditis
- normal variant - 'high take-off'
- left ventricular aneurysm
- Prinzmetal's angina (coronary artery spasm)
- rare: subarachnoid haemorrhage, part of spectrum of changes in hyperkalaemia

Cardiac action potential

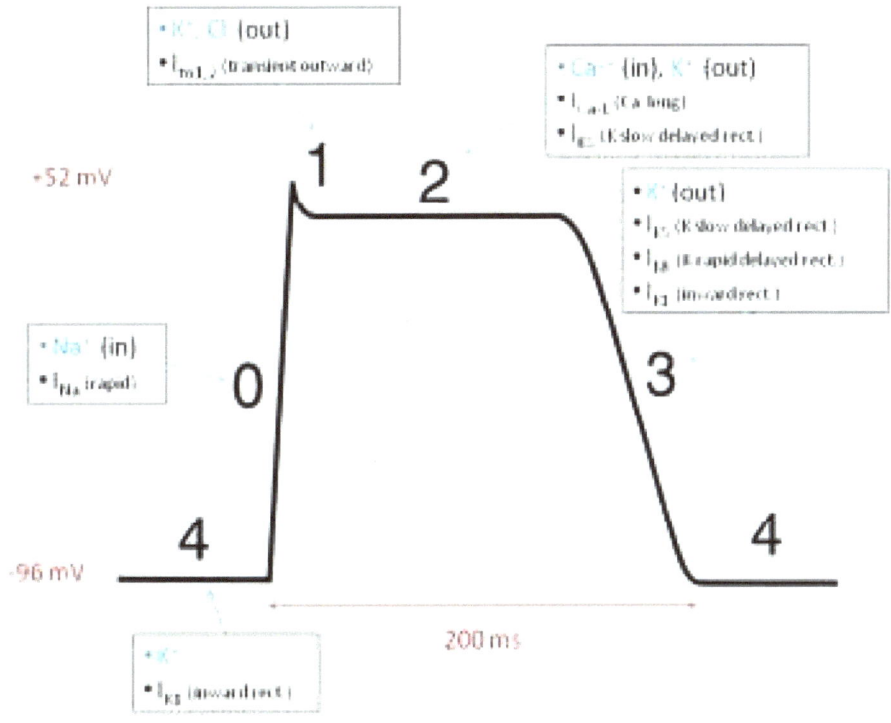

Phase	Description	Mechanism
0	Rapid depolarization	Rapid sodium influx. These channels automatically deactivate after a few ms
1	Early repolarisation	Efflux of potassium
2	Plateau	Slow influx of calcium
3	Final repolarisation	Efflux of potassium
4	Restoration of ionic concentrations	Resting potential is restored by Na$^+$/K$^+$ ATPase. There is slow entry of Na$^+$ into the cell decreasing the potential difference until the threshold potential is reached, triggering a new action potential

NB cardiac muscle remains contracted 10-15 times longer than skeletal muscle

Conduction velocity

Site	Speed
Atrial conduction	Spreads along ordinary atrial myocardial fibres at 1 m/sec
AV node conduction	0.05 m/sec
Ventricular conduction	Purkinje fibres are of large diameter and achieve velocities of 2-4 m/sec (this allows a rapid and coordinated contraction of the ventricles

Multifocal atrial tachycardia (MAT)

- May be defined as a irregular cardiac rhythm caused by at least three different sites in the atria, which may be demonstrated by morphologically distinctive P waves.
- It is more common in elderly patients with chronic lung disease, for example COPD

Management:
- ✓ correction of hypoxia and electrolyte disturbances
- ✓ rate-limiting calcium channel blockers are often used first-line
- ✓ cardioversion and digoxin are not useful in the management of MAT

Supraventricular tachycardia

- Whilst strictly speaking the term supraventricular tachycardia (SVT) refers to any tachycardia that is not ventricular in origin the term is generally used in the context of paroxysmal SVT.
- Episodes are characterised by the sudden onset of a narrow complex tachycardia, typically an atrioventricular nodal re-entry tachycardia (AVNRT).
- Other causes include:
  - ✓ atrioventricular re-entry tachycardias (AVRT) and

- ✓ junctional tachycardias:

Acute management:
- ➢ vagal manoeuvres: e.g. Valsalva manoeuvre
- ➢ intravenous adenosine
    - ✓ 6mg → 12mg → 12mg
    - ✓ contraindicated in asthmatics - verapamil is a preferable option
- ➢ electrical cardioversion

Prevention of episodes:
- beta-blockers
- radio-frequency ablation

Wolff-Parkinson White (WPW)

- WPW is caused by a congenital accessory conducting pathway between the atria and ventricles leading to atrioventricular re-entry tachycardia (AVRT).
- As the accessory pathway does not slow conduction AF can degenerate rapidly to VF

Possible ECG features include:
- short PR interval
- wide QRS complexes with a slurred upstroke - 'delta wave'
- left axis deviation if right-sided accessory pathway*
- right axis deviation if left-sided accessory pathway*

*in the majority of cases, or in a question without qualification, Wolff-Parkinson-White syndrome is associated with left axis deviation

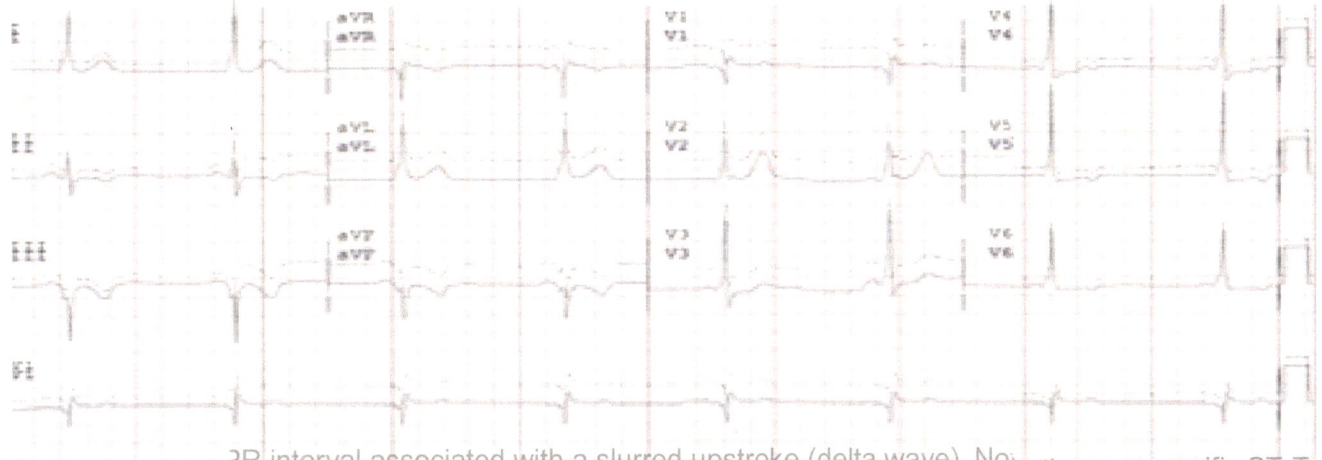

ECG showing short PR interval associated with a slurred upstroke (delta wave). Note the non-specific ST-T changes which are common in WPW and may be mistaken for ischaemia. The left axis deviation means that this is type B WPW, implying a right-sided pathway

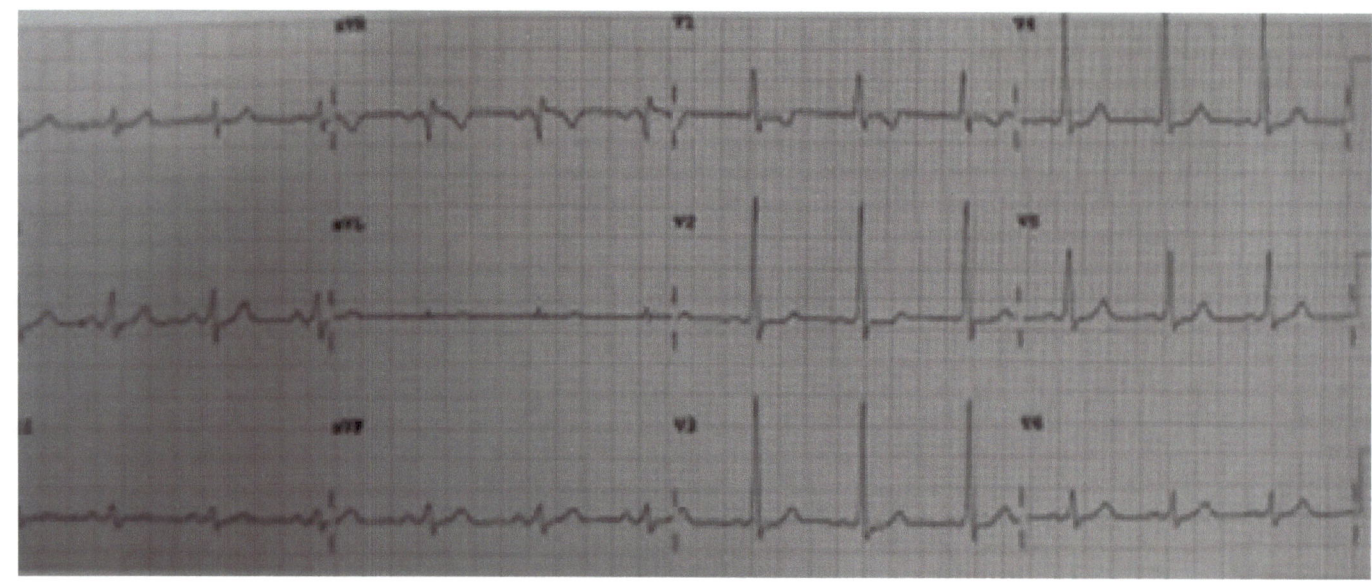

Further example showing a characteristic delta wave

Differentiating between type A and type B
- type A (left-sided pathway): dominant R wave in V1
- type B (right-sided pathway): no dominant R wave in V1

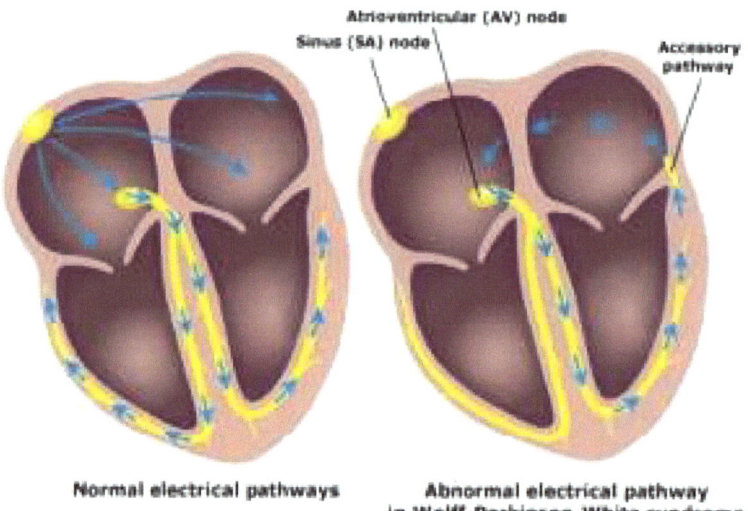

Associations of WPW
- HOCM
- mitral valve prolapse
- Ebstein's anomaly
- thyrotoxicosis
- secundum ASD

Management:
> definitive treatment: radiofrequency ablation of the accessory pathway

- medical therapy: sotalol**, amiodarone, flecainide

**sotalol should be avoided if there is coexistent atrial fibrillation as prolonging the refractory period at the AV node may increase the rate of transmission through the accessory pathway, increasing the ventricular rate and potentially deteriorating into ventricular fibrillation

Atrial fibrillation:

Classification:

- An attempt was made in the joint American Heart Association (AHA), American College of Cardiology (ACC) and European Society of Cardiology (ESC) 2012 guidelines to simplify and clarify the classification of atrial fibrillation (AF).
- It is recommended that AF be classified into 3 patterns:

  - first detected episode (irrespective of whether it is symptomatic or self-terminating)
  - Recurrent episodes:
    - When a patient has 2 or more episodes of AF.
    - If episodes of AF terminate spontaneously then the term **paroxysmal AF** is used. Such episodes last less than 7 days (typically < 24 hours).
    - If the arrhythmia is not self-terminating then the term **persistent AF** is used. Such episodes usually last greater than 7 days
  - In **permanent AF** there is continuous atrial fibrillation which cannot be cardioverted or if attempts to do so are deemed inappropriate. Treatment goals are therefore rate control and anticoagulation if appropriate

Atrial fibrillation: post-stroke

- NICE issued guidelines on atrial fibrillation (AF) in 2006.
- They included advice on the management of patients with AF who develop a stroke or transient-ischaemic attack (TIA).

Recommendations include:
- Following a stroke or TIA warfarin should be given as the anticoagulant of choice.
- Aspirin/dipyridamole should only be given if needed for the treatment of other comorbidities
- In acute stroke patients, in the absence of haemorrhage, anticoagulation therapy should be commenced after 2 weeks.
- If imaging shows a very large cerebral infarction then the initiation of anticoagulation should be delayed

Atrial fibrillation: rate control and maintenance of sinus rhythm

- The Royal College of Physicians and NICE published guidelines on the management of atrial fibrillation (AF) in 2006.
- The following is also based on the joint American Heart Association (AHA), American College of Cardiology (ACC) and European Society of Cardiology (ESC) 2012 guidelines

Agents used to control rate in patients with atrial fibrillation
- beta-blockers
- calcium channel blockers
- digoxin (not considered first-line anymore as they are less effective at controlling the heart rate during exercise. However, they are the preferred choice if the patient has coexistent heart failure)

Agents used to maintain sinus rhythm in patients with a history of atrial fibrillation
- sotalol
- amiodarone
- flecainide
- others (less commonly used in UK): disopyramide, dofetilide, procainamide, propafenone, quinidine

The table below indicates some of the factors which may be considered when considering either a rate control or rhythm control strategy

Factors favouring rate control	Factors favouring rhythm control
- Older than 65 years - History of ischaemic heart disease	- Younger than 65 years - Symptomatic - First presentation - Lone AF or AF secondary to a corrected precipitant (e.g. Alcohol) - Congestive heart failure

Pharmacological cardioversion

Agents with proven efficacy in the pharmacological cardioversion of atrial fibrillation:
- Amiodarone (if structural heart disease)
- flecainide (if no structural heart disease)
- others (less commonly used in UK): quinidine, dofetilide, ibutilide, propafenone

Less effective agents:
- beta-blockers (including sotalol)
- calcium channel blockers
- digoxin

- disopyramide
- procainamide

Atrial fibrillation: cardioversion

Onset < 48 hours

- If the atrial fibrillation (AF) is definitely of less than 48 hours onset patients should be heparinised.
- Patients who have risk factors for ischaemic stroke should be put on lifelong oral anticoagulation.
- Otherwise, patients may be cardioverted using either:
  - electrical - 'DC cardioversion'
  - pharmacology - amiodarone if structural heart disease, flecainide in those without structural heart disease
- Following electrical cardioversion if AF is confirmed as being less than 48 hours duration then further anticoagulation is unnecessary

Onset > 48 hours

- If the patient has been in AF for more than 48 hours then anticoagulation should be given for at least 3 weeks prior to cardioversion.
- An alternative strategy is to perform a transoesophageal echo (TOE) to exclude a left atrial appendage (LAA) thrombus.
- If excluded patients may be heparinised and cardioverted immediately.
- If there is a high risk of cardioversion failure (e.g. Previous failure or AF recurrence) then it is recommend to have at least 4 weeks amiodarone or sotalol prior to electrical cardioversion
- Following electrical cardioversion patients should be anticoagulated for at least 4 weeks. After this time decisions about anticoagulation should be taken on an individual basis depending on the risk of recurrence

Paradoxical embolisation

- For a right-sided thrombus (e.g. DVT) to cause a left-sided embolism (e.g. stroke) it must obviously pass from the right-to-left side of the heart
- The following cardiac lesions may cause such events:

  - patent foramen ovale: present in around 20% of the population
  - atrial septal defect: a much less common cause

Antiarrhythmics: Vaughan Williams classification

- The Vaughan Williams classification of antiarrhythmics is still widely used although it should be noted that a number of common drugs are not included in the classification e.g. adenosine, atropine, digoxin and magnesium
AP = action potential

Class	Examples	Mechanism of action	Notes
Ia	Quinidine Procainamide Disopyramide	1) Block sodium channels 2) Increases AP duration	- Quinidine toxicity causes cinchonism (headache, tinnitus, thrombocytopaenia) - Procainamide may cause drug-induced lupus
Ib	Lidocaine Mexiletine Tocainide	1) Block sodium channels 2) Decreases AP duration	
Ic	Flecainide Encainide Propafenone	1) Block sodium channels 2) No effect on AP duration	
II	Propranolol Atenolol Bisoprolol Metoprolol	Beta-adrenoceptor antagonists	
III	Amiodarone Sotalol Ibutilide Bretylium	Block potassium channels	
IV	Verapamil Diltiazem	Calcium channel blockers	

Flecainide

- Flecainide is a Vaughan Williams class 1c antiarrhythmic.
- It slows conduction of the action potential by acting as a potent sodium channel blocker.
- This may be reflected by widening of the QRS complex and prolongation of the PR interval
- The Cardiac Arrhythmia Suppression Trial (CAST, 1989) investigated the use of agents to treat asymptomatic or mildly symptomatic premature ventricular complexes (PVCs) post myocardial infarction. The hypothesis was that this would reduce deaths from ventricular arrhythmias. Flecainide was actually shown to increase mortality post myocardial infarction and is therefore contraindicated in this situation

Indications:
- atrial fibrillation
- SVT associated with accessory pathway e.g. Wolf-Parkinson-White syndrome

Adverse effects:
1) negatively inotropic
2) bradycardia
3) proarrhythmic
4) oral paraesthesia
5) visual disturbances

Amiodarone

- Amiodarone is a class III antiarrhythmic agent used in the treatment of atrial, nodal and ventricular tachycardias.
- The main mechanism of action is by blocking potassium channels which inhibits repolarisation and hence prolongs the action potential.
- Amiodarone also has other actions such as blocking sodium channels (a class I effect)
- The use of amiodarone is limited by a number of factors:
  - long half-life (20-100 days)
  - should ideally be given into central veins (causes thrombophlebitis)
  - has proarrhythmic effects due to lengthening of the QT interval
  - interacts with drugs commonly used concurrently e.g. Decreases metabolism of warfarin
  - numerous long-term adverse effects (see below)

Amiodarone adverse effects:

1) thyroid dysfunction: both hypothyroidism and hyperthyroidism
2) corneal deposits: present in most patients, rarely interfere with vision, usually reversible on withdrawal of drug
3) photosensitivity
4) pulmonary fibrosis/pneumonitis
5) liver cirrhosis/hepatitis
6) peripheral neuropathy, myopathy

'slate-grey' appearance
7) prolonged QT interval
8) thrombophlebitis and injection site reactions
9) bradycardia

Important drug interactions of amiodarone include:
1) decreased metabolism of warfarin; therefore increased INR
2) increased digoxin levels

Monitoring of patients taking amiodarone
- TFT, LFT, U&E, CXR prior to treatment
- TFT, LFT every 6 months

Amiodarone and the thyroid gland

Around 1 in 6 patients taking amiodarone develop thyroid dysfunction

A) **Amiodarone-induced hypothyroidism:** (AIH)
- The pathophysiology of amiodarone-induced hypothyroidism (AIH) is thought to be due to the high iodine content of amiodarone causing a Wolff-Chaikoff effect*
- Amiodarone may be continued if this is desirable

*an autoregulatory phenomenon where thyroxine formation is inhibited due to high levels of circulating iodide

B) **Amiodarone-induced thyrotoxicosis** (AIT)

Amiodarone-induced thyrotoxicosis (AIT) may be divided into two types:

	AIT type 1	AIT type 2
Pathophysiology	Excess iodine-induced thyroid hormone synthesis	Amiodarone-related destructive thyroiditis
Goitre	Present	Absent
Management	Carbimazole or potassium perchlorate	Corticosteroids

Unlike in AIH, amiodarone should be stopped if possible in patients who develop AIT

Adenosine

- The effects of adenosine are:
  - ⇒ Enhanced by dipyridamole (anti-platelet agent) and
  - ⇒ blocked by theophyllines
- It should be avoided in asthmatics due to possible bronchospasm.

Mechanism of action:
1) causes transient heart block in the AV node
2) agonist of the A1 receptor which inhibits adenylyl cyclase thus reducing cAMP and causing hyperpolarization by increasing outward potassium flux
3) adenosine has a very short half-life of about 8-10 seconds

Adverse effects:
1) chest pain
2) bronchospasm
3) can enhance conduction down accessory pathways, resulting in increased ventricular rate (e.g. WPW syndrome)

Adrenaline

Adrenaline is a sympathomimetic amine with both alpha and beta adrenergic stimulating properties

Indications:
- anaphylaxis
- cardiac arrest

Recommend Adult Life Support (ALS) adrenaline doses:
1) anaphylaxis: 0.5ml 1:1,000 IM
2) cardiac arrest:
   - ⇒ 1ml of 1:1000 IV
   - ⇒ 10ml 1:10,000 IV

Management of accidental injection:
- local infiltration of phentolamine

Adrenoceptor antagonists

Alpha antagonists
- alpha-1: doxazosin
- alpha-1a: tamsulosin - acts mainly on urogenital tract
- alpha-2: yohimbine

- non-selective: phenoxybenzamine (previously used in peripheral arterial disease)

Beta antagonists
- beta-1: atenolol
- non-selective: propranolol

Mixed alpha and beta antagonists
- Carvedilol and labetalol

Atrial fibrillation: anticoagulation

- The European Society of Cardiology published updated guidelines on the management of atrial fibrillation in 2012.
- They suggest using the **CHA$_2$DS$_2$-VASc** score to determine the most appropriate anticoagulation strategy. This scoring system superceded the CHADS$_2$ score.

	Risk factor	Points
C	Congestive heart failure	1
H	Hypertension (or treated hypertension)	1
A$_2$	Age >= 75 years	2
	Age 65-74 years	1
D	Diabetes	1
S$_2$	Prior Stroke or TIA	2
V	Vascular disease (including ischaemic heart disease and peripheral arterial disease)	1
S	Sex (female)	1

The table below shows a suggested anticoagulation strategy based on the score:

Score	Anticoagulation
0	No treatment
1	Males: Consider anticoagulation Females: No treatment
2 or more	Offer anticoagulation

- Doctors have always thought carefully about the risk/benefit profile of starting someone on warfarin.
- A history of falls, old age, alcohol excess and a history of previous bleeding are common things that make us consider whether warfarinisation is in the best interests of the patient.
- NICE now recommend we formalise this risk assessment using the HASBLED scoring system.

	Risk factor	Points
H	Hypertension, uncontrolled, systolic BP > 160 mmHg	1
A	Abnormal renal function (dialysis or creatinine > 200) Or Abnormal liver function (cirrhosis, bilirubin > 2 times normal, ALT/AST/ALP > 3 times normal	1 for any renal abnormalities 1 for any liver abnormalities
S	Stroke, history of	1
B	Bleeding, history of bleeding or tendency to bleed	1
L	Labile INRs (unstable/high INRs, time in therapeutic range < 60%)	1
E	Elderly (> 65 years)	1
D	Drugs Predisposing to Bleeding (Antiplatelet agents, NSAIDs) Or Alcohol Use (>8 drinks/week)	1 for drugs 1 for alcohol

Atrial flutter

Atrial flutter is a form of supraventricular tachycardia characterised by a succession of rapid atrial depolarisation waves.

ECG findings
- 'sawtooth' appearance
- as the underlying atrial rate is often around 300/min the ventricular or heart rate is dependent on the degree of AV block. For example if there is 2:1 block the ventricular rate will be 150/min
- flutter waves may be visible following carotid sinus massage or adenosine

Management:
- is similar to that of atrial fibrillation although medication may be less effective
- atrial flutter is more sensitive to cardioversion however so lower energy levels may be used
- radiofrequency ablation of the tricuspid valve isthmus is curative for most patients

Long QT syndrome

- Long QT syndrome (LQTS) is an inherited condition associated with delayed repolarization of the ventricles.
- It is important to recognise as it may lead to ventricular tachycardia and can therefore cause collapse/sudden death.
- The most common variants of LQTS (LQT1 & LQT2) are caused by defects in the alpha subunit of the slow delayed rectifier potassium channel.
- A normal corrected QT interval is less than 430 ms in males and 450 ms in females.

Causes of a prolonged QT interval:

Congenital

Jervell-Lange-Nielsen syndrome (includes deafness and is due to an abnormal potassium channel)

Romano-Ward syndrome (no deafness)

Drugs*
- amiodarone, sotalol, class 1a antiarrhythmic drugs
- tricyclic antidepressants,
- selective serotonin reuptake inhibitors (especially citalopram)
- haloperidol
- methadone
- chloroquine
- terfenadine**
- erythromycin

Other
- electrolyte: hypocalcaemia, hypokalaemia, hypomagnesaemia
- hypothermia
- subarachnoid haemorrhage
- acute myocardial infarction
- myocarditis

Features:
- may be picked up on routine ECG or following family screening
- sudden cardiac death
- **Long QT1:** Usually associated with exertional syncope, often swimming
- **Long QT2:** Often associated with syncope occurring following emotional stress, exercise or auditory stimuli
- **Long QT3:** events often occur at night or at rest

Management:
- avoid drugs which prolong the QT interval and other precipitants if appropriate (e.g. strenuous exercise)
- beta-blockers***
- implantable cardioverter defibrillators in high risk cases

*the usual mechanism by which drugs prolong the QT interval is blockage of potassium channels.
**a non-sedating antihistamine are classic cause of prolonged QT in a patient, especially if also taking P450 enzyme inhibitor, e.g. Patient with a cold takes terfenadine and erythromycin at the same time
***note sotalol may exacerbate long QT syndrome

Broad complex tachycardia

- Whilst a broad complex tachycardia may result from a supraventricular rhythm with aberrant conduction, the European Resuscitation Council advise that in a peri-arrest situation it is assumed to be ventricular in origin
- Features suggesting VT rather than SVT with aberrant conduction

- AV dissociation
- fusion or capture beats
- positive QRS concordance in chest leads
- marked left axis deviation
- history of IHD
- lack of response to adenosine or carotid sinus massage
- QRS > 160 ms

Ventricular tachycardia

- Ventricular tachycardia (VT) is broad-complex tachycardia originating from a ventricular ectopic focus.
- It has the potential to precipitate ventricular fibrillation and hence requires urgent treatment.
- There are two main types of VT:

  - Monomorphic VT: most commonly caused by myocardial infarction
  - Polymorphic VT: A subtype of polymorphic VT is torsades de pointes which is precipitated by prolongation of the QT interval.

Management:
- If the patient has adverse signs (systolic BP < 90 mmHg, chest pain, heart failure or rate > 150 beats/min) then immediate cardioversion is indicated.
- In the absence of such signs antiarrhythmics may be used. If these fail, then electrical cardioversion may be needed with synchronised DC shocks

Drug therapy:
- amiodarone: ideally administered through a central line
- lidocaine: use with caution in severe left ventricular impairment
- procainamide

Verapamil should NOT be used in VT

If drug therapy fails:
- electrophysiological study (EPS)
- implant able cardioverter-defibrillator (ICD) - this is particularly indicated in patients with significantly impaired LV function

Torsades de pointes

- Torsades de pointes ('twisting of the points') is a rare arrhythmia associated with a long QT interval.
- It may deteriorate into ventricular fibrillation and hence lead to sudden death

Causes of long QT interval:

- congenital: Jervell-Lange-Nielsen syndrome, Romano-Ward syndrome
- antiarrhythmics: amiodarone, sotalol, class 1a antiarrhythmic drugs
- tricyclic antidepressants
- antipsychotics
- chloroquine
- terfenadine
- erythromycin
- electrolyte: hypocalcaemia, hypokalaemia, hypomagnesaemia
- myocarditis
- hypothermia
- subarachnoid haemorrhage

Management:
- IV magnesium sulphate

ECG: hypothermia

The following ECG changes may be seen in hypothermia

- bradycardia
- 'J' wave - small hump at the end of the QRS complex
- first degree heart block
- long QT interval
- atrial and ventricular arrhythmias

ECG: left bundle branch block

The diagram below shows the typical features of left bundle branch block (LBBB):

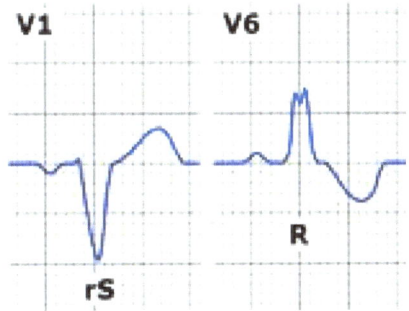

One of the most common ways to remember the difference between LBBB and RBBB is WiLLiaM MaRRoW

- in LBBB there is a 'W' in V1 and a 'M' in V6
- in RBBB there is a 'M' in V1 and a 'W' in V6

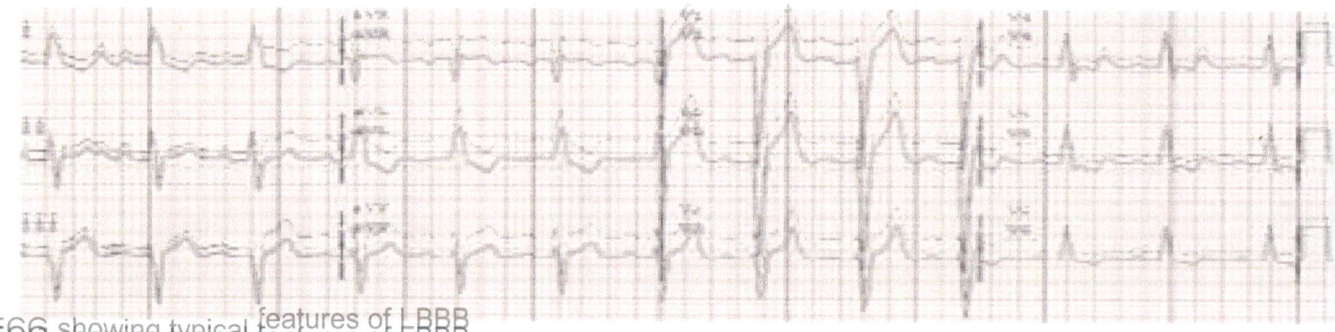

ECG showing typical features of LBBB

Causes of LBBB:
- ischaemic heart disease
- hypertension
- aortic stenosis
- cardiomyopathy
- rare: idiopathic fibrosis, digoxin toxicity, hyperkalaemia

Types of heart block:

First degree heart block:
- PR interval > 0.2 seconds

Second degree heart block:
- **Type 1 (Mobitz I; Wenckebach):** progressive prolongation of the PR interval until a dropped beat occurs
- **Type 2 (Mobitz II):** PR interval is constant but the P wave is often not followed by a QRS complex

Third degree (complete) heart block
- there is no association between the P waves and QRS complexes

Complete heart block

Features:
- syncope
- heart failure
- regular bradycardia (30-50 bpm)
- wide pulse pressure
- JVP: cannon waves in neck
- variable intensity of S1

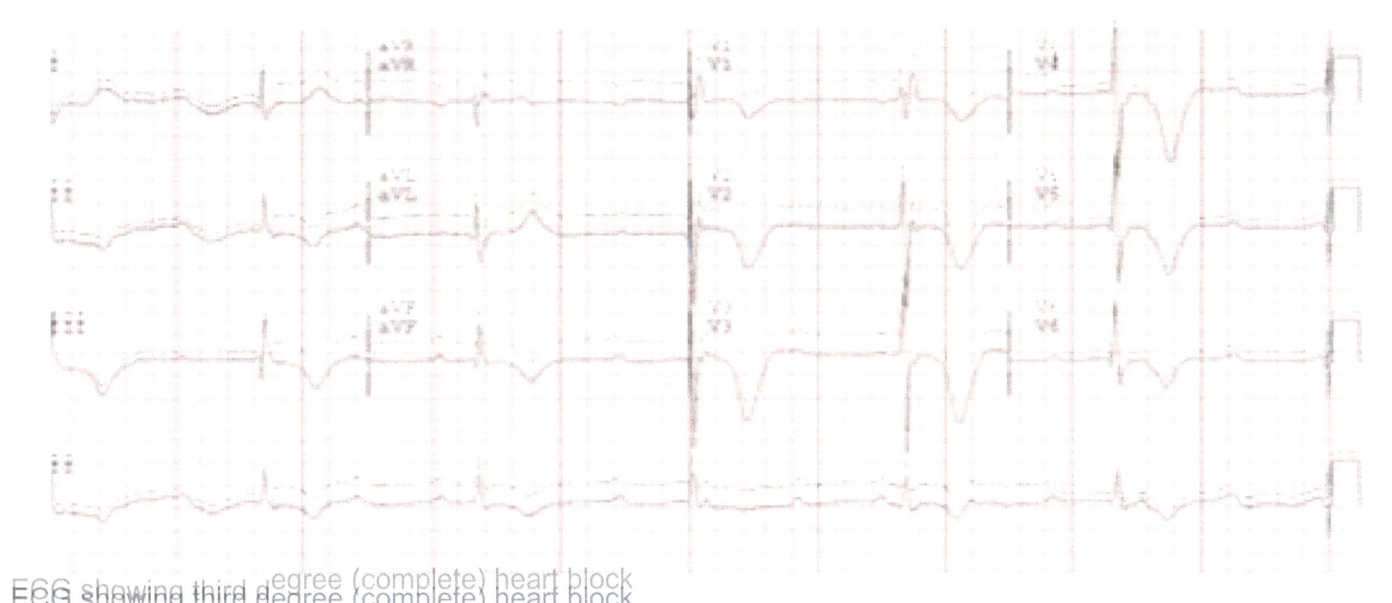
ECG showing third degree (complete) heart block

Peri-arrest rhythms:

Bradycardia

The 2010 Resuscitation Council (UK) guidelines emphasise that the management of bradycardia depends on:

1. Identifying the presence of signs indicating haemodynamic compromise = 'adverse signs'
2. Identifying the potential risk of asystole

Adverse signs

The following factors indicate haemodynamic compromise and hence the need for treatment:

1) shock: hypotension (systolic blood pressure < 90 mmHg); pallor; sweating; cold; clammy extremities; confusion or impaired consciousness
2) syncope
3) myocardial ischaemia
4) heart failure

- Atropine is the first line treatment in this situation.
- If this fails to work, or there is the potential risk of asystole then transvenous pacing is indicated

Potential risk of asystole:

The following indicate a potential risk of asystole and hence the need for treatment with transvenous pacing:

- complete heart block with broad complex QRS
- recent asystole
- Mobitz type II AV block
- ventricular pause > 3 seconds

If there is a delay in the provision of transvenous pacing the following interventions may be used:

- atropine, up to maximum of 3mg
- transcutaneous pacing
- adrenaline infusion titrated to response

Peri-arrest tachycardia

- The 2010 Resuscitation Council (UK) guidelines have simplified the advice given for the management of peri-arrest tachycardias.
- Separate algorithms for the management of broad-complex tachycardia, narrow complex tachycardia and atrial fibrillation have been replaced by one unified treatment algorithm
- Following basic ABC assessment, patients are classified as being stable or unstable according to the presence of any adverse signs (as above)
- If any of the above adverse signs are present then **synchronised DC shocks** should be given
- Treatment following this is given according to whether the QRS complex is narrow or broad and whether the rhythm is regular or irregular.
- The full treatment algorithm can be found at the Resuscitation Council website, below is a very limited summary:

1) **Broad-complex tachycardia**
   Regular:
   - assume ventricular tachycardia (unless previously confirmed SVT with bundle branch block)
   - loading dose of amiodarone followed by 24 hour infusion

   Irregular:
   1. AF with bundle branch block - treat as for narrow complex tachycardia.
   2. Polymorphic VT (e.g. Torsade de pointes) - IV magnesium

2) **Narrow-complex tachycardia**
   Regular:
   - vagal manoeuvres followed by IV adenosine
   - if above unsuccessful consider diagnosis of atrial flutter and control rate (e.g. Beta-blockers)

Irregular:
- probable atrial fibrillation
- if onset < 48 hr consider electrical or chemical cardioversion
- rate control (e.g. Beta-blocker or digoxin) and anticoagulation

Pacemakers:
Temporary:
Indications for a temporary pacemaker

- symptomatic/haemodynamically unstable bradycardia, not responding to atropine
- post-ANTERIOR MI: type 2 or complete heart block*
- trifascicular block prior to surgery

*post-INFERIOR MI complete heart block is common and can be managed conservatively if asymptomatic and haemodynamically stable

Implantable cardiac defibrillators
Indications
- long QT syndrome
- hypertrophic obstructive cardiomyopathy
- previous cardiac arrest due to VT/VF
- previous myocardial infarction with non-sustained VT on 24 hr monitoring,
- inducible VT on electrophysiology testing and ejection fraction < 35%
- Brugada syndrome

ECG: axis deviation
Causes of left axis deviation (LAD):
- left anterior hemiblock
- left bundle branch block
- Wolff-Parkinson-White syndrome* - right-sided accessory pathway
- hyperkalaemia
- congenital: ostium primum ASD, tricuspid atresia
- minor LAD in obese people

Causes of right axis deviation (RAD):
- right ventricular hypertrophy
- chronic lung disease → cor pulmonale
- pulmonary embolism
- left posterior hemiblock

- ostium secundum ASD
- Wolff-Parkinson-White syndrome* - left-sided accessory pathway
- normal in infant ≤ 1 years old
- minor RAD in tall people

*in the majority of cases, or in a question without qualification, Wolff-Parkinson-White syndrome is associated with left axis deviation

Coarctation of the aorta

- Coarctation of the aorta describes a congenital narrowing of the descending aorta.
- more common in males (despite association with Turner's syndrome)

Features:
- infancy: heart failure
- adult: hypertension
- radio-femoral delay
- mid systolic murmur, maximal over back
- apical click from the aortic valve
- notching of the inferior border of the ribs (due to collateral vessels) is not seen in young children

Associations:
- Turner's syndrome
- bicuspid aortic valve
- berry aneurysms
- neurofibromatosis

Aortic dissection

Stanford classification:
- type A = ascending aorta, 2/3 of cases
- type B = descending aorta, distal to left subclavian origin, 1/3 of cases

DeBakey classification:
- type I = originates in ascending aorta, propagates to at least the aortic arch and possibly beyond it distally
- type II = originates in and is confined to the ascending aorta
- type III = originates in descending aorta, rarely extends proximally but will extend distally

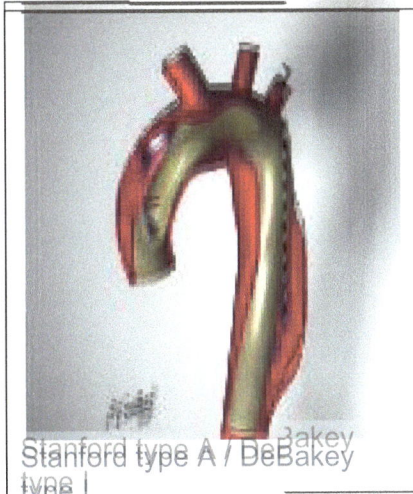 Stanford type A / DeBakey type I
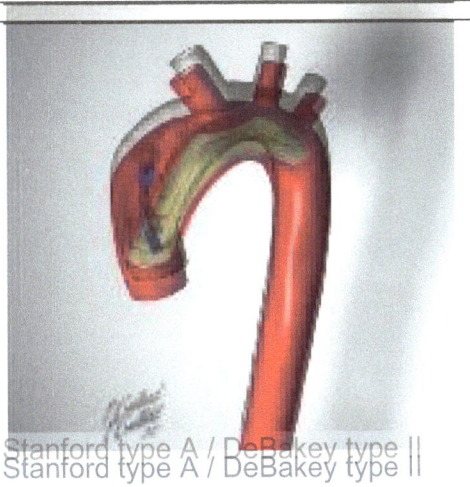 Stanford type A / DeBakey type II
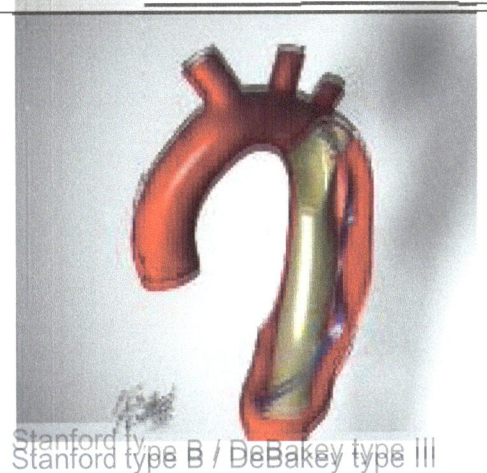 Stanford type B / DeBakey type III

Associations:
- hypertension
- trauma
- bicuspid aortic valve
- collagens: Marfan's syndrome, Ehlers-Danlos syndrome
- Turner's and Noonan's syndrome
- pregnancy
- syphilis

Complications of backward tear:
- aortic incompetence/regurgitation
- MI: inferior pattern often seen due to right coronary involvement

Complications of forward tear

- unequal arm pulses and BP
- stroke
- renal failure

Aortic dissection management:

Type A
- surgical management; but blood pressure should be controlled to a target systolic of 100-120 mmHg whilst awaiting intervention

Type B*
- conservative management
- bed rest
- reduce blood pressure IV labetalol to prevent progression

*endovascular repair of type B aortic dissection may have a role in the future

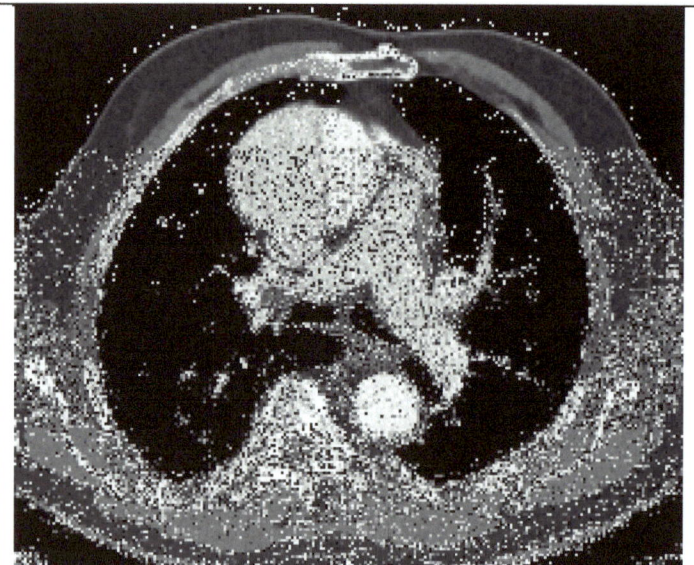

An intraluminal tear has formed a 'flap' that can be clearly seen in the ascending aorta. This is a Stanford type A dissection

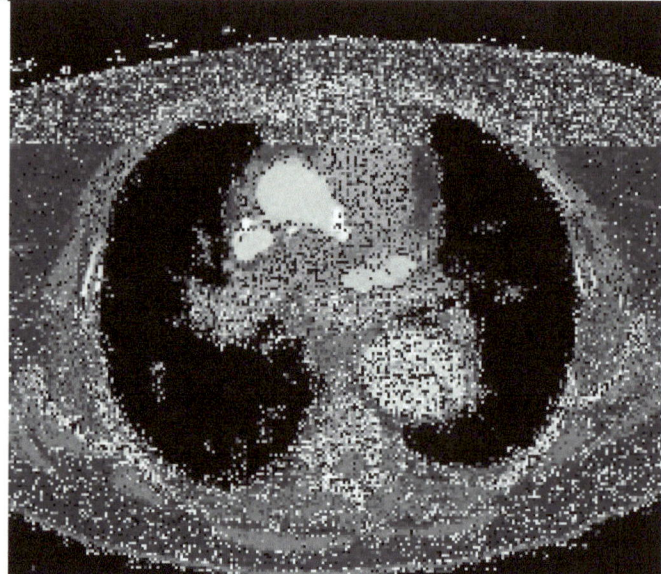

Stanford type B dissection, seen in the descending aorta

Pulmonary arterial hypertension:

PAH may be defined as a sustained elevation in mean pulmonary arterial pressure of greater than 25 mmHg at rest or 30 mmHg after exercise.

Features:
- exertional dyspnoea is the most frequent symptom
- chest pain and syncope may also occur
- loud P2
- left parasternal heave (due to right ventricular hypertrophy)

Causes and classification:

PAH has recently been reclassified by the WHO:

Group 1: Pulmonary arterial hypertension (PAH)
- idiopathic*
- familial
- associated conditions:
    - ✓ Collagen vascular disease,
    - ✓ congenital heart disease with systemic to pulmonary shunts,
    - ✓ HIV**,
    - ✓ drugs and toxins,

          ✓ sickle cell disease
    - persistent pulmonary hypertension of the newborn

*previously termed primary pulmonary hypertension
**the mechanism by which HIV infection produces pulmonary hypertension remains unknown

Group 2: Pulmonary hypertension with left heart disease
- left-sided atrial, ventricular or valvular disease such as left ventricular systolic and diastolic dysfunction, mitral stenosis and mitral regurgitation

Group 3: Pulmonary hypertension secondary to lung disease/hypoxia
- COPD
- interstitial lung disease
- sleep apnoea
- high altitude

Group 4: Pulmonary hypertension due to thromboembolic disease

Group 5: Miscellaneous conditions
- lymphangiomatosis e.g. secondary to carcinomatosis or sarcoidosis

Pulmonary arterial hypertension management
- Management should first involve treating any underlying conditions, for example with anticoagulants or oxygen.
- Following this, it has now been shown that **acute vasodilator testing** is central to deciding on the appropriate management strategy.
- Acute vasodilator testing:
    - ✓ Aims to decide which patients show a significant fall in pulmonary arterial pressure following the administration of vasodilators such as **intravenous epoprostenol** or **inhaled nitric oxide**
    - ✓ If there is a positive response to acute vasodilator testing: treat with oral calcium channel blockers
    - ✓ If there is a negative response to acute vasodilator testing:
        - **prostacyclin analogues**: treprostinil, iloprost
        - **endothelin receptor antagonists**: bosentan
        - **phosphodiesterase inhibitors**: sildenafil

Primary pulmonary hypertension
- The classification of pulmonary hypertension is currently changing with the term idiopathic pulmonary arterial hypertension (IPAH) becoming more widely used
-

- Primary pulmonary hypertension (PPH; now IPAH)

  - pulmonary arterial pressure > 25 mmHg at rest; > 30mmHg with exercise
  - PPH is diagnosed when no underlying cause can be found
  - around 10% of cases are familial: autosomal dominant
  - endothelin thought to play a key role in pathogenesis
  - associated with HIV; cocaine and anorexigens (e.g. fenfluramine)

Features:
- more common in females; typically presents at 20-40 years old
- progressive SOB
- cyanosis
- right ventricular heave; loud P2; raised JVP with prominent 'a' waves, tricuspid regurgitation

Investigation:
- echocardiography

Management:
- diuretics if right heart failure
- anticoagulation
- vasodilator therapy: calcium channel blocker; IV prostaglandins; bosentan: endothelin-1 receptor antagonist
- heart-lung transplant

Pericarditis

Pericarditis is one of the differentials of any patient presenting with chest pain.

Features:
- Chest pain: may be pleuritic. Is often relieved by sitting forwards
- other symptoms include non-productive cough, dyspnoea and flu-like symptoms
- pericardial rub
- tachypnoea
- tachycardia

Causes:
- viral infections (Coxsackie)
- tuberculosis
- uraemia (causes 'fibrinous' pericarditis)
- trauma
- post-myocardial infarction; Dressler's syndrome
- connective tissue disease
- hypothyroidism

ECG changes

- widespread 'saddle-shaped' ST elevation
- PR depression: most specific ECG marker for pericarditis

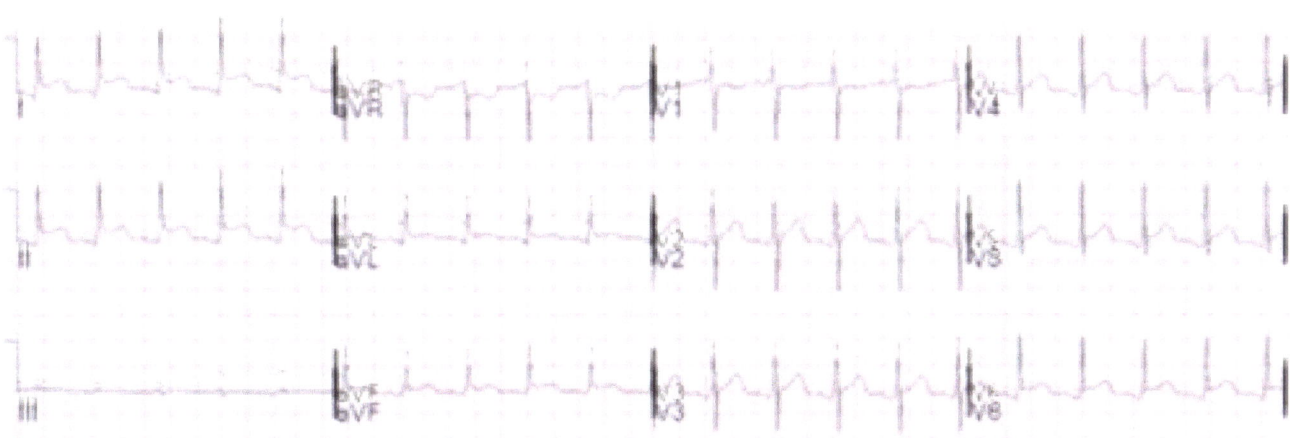

ECG showing pericarditis. Note the widespread nature of the ST elevation and the PR depression

Rheumatic fever: criteria

- Rheumatic fever develops following an immunological reaction to recent (2-6 weeks ago) Streptococcus pyogenes infection.
- Diagnosis is based on evidence of recent streptococcal infection accompanied by:

  - 2 major criteria
  - 1 major with 2 minor criteria

Evidence of recent streptococcal infection:
- history of scarlet fever
- ASOT > 200iu/mL
- positive throat swab
- increase in DNase B titre

Major criteria:
- erythema marginatum
- Sydenham's chorea
- polyarthritis
- carditis (endo-, myo- or peri-)
- subcutaneous nodules

Minor criteria:
- raised ESR or CRP

- pyrexia
- arthralgia (not if arthritis a major criteria)
- prolonged PR interval

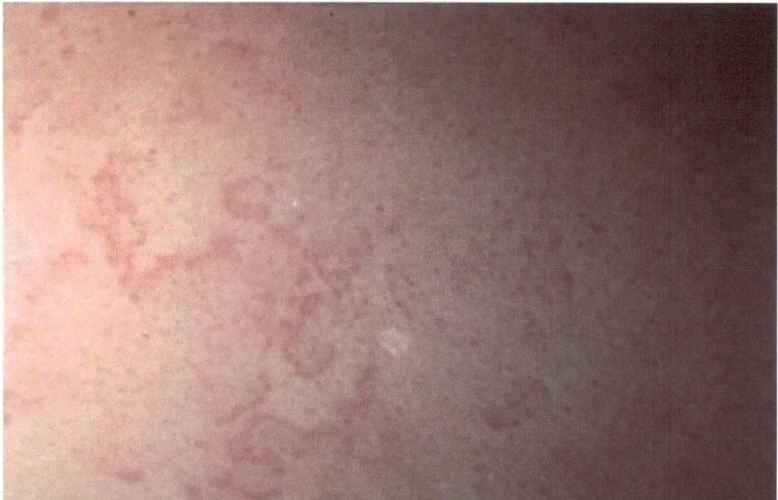

Erythema marginatum is seen in around 10% of children with rheumatic fever. It is rare in adults

Infective endocarditis

- The strongest risk factor for developing infective endocarditis is a previous episode of endocarditis.
- The following types of patients are affected:
    - ✓ previously normal valves (50%, typically acute presentation)
    - ✓ Rheumatic valve disease (30%)
    - ✓ prosthetic valves
    - ✓ congenital heart defects
    - ✓ intravenous drug users (IVDUs, e.g. Typically causing tricuspid lesion)

Causes:
- Streptococcus viridans (most common cause - 40-50%)
- Staphylococcus epidermidis (especially prosthetic valves)
- Staphylococcus aureus (especially acute presentation, IVDUs)
- Streptococcus bovis is associated with colorectal cancer
- Streptococcus mitis (viridans streptococcus): following dental work
- non-infective: systemic lupus erythematosus (Libman-Sacks), malignancy: marantic endocarditis

Culture negative causes:
- prior antibiotic therapy
- Coxiella burnetii
- Bartonella

- Brucella
- HACEK: Haemophilus, Actinobacillus, Cardiobacterium, Eikenella, Kingella)

- Following prosthetic valve surgery Staphylococcus epidermidis is the most common organism in the first 2 months and is usually the result of perioperative contamination.
- After 2 months the spectrum of organisms which cause endocarditis return to normal, except with a slight increase in Staph. aureus infections

Infective endocarditis: Modified Duke Criteria

Infective endocarditis diagnosed if:
- pathological criteria positive, or
- 2 major criteria, or
- 1 major and 3 minor criteria, or
- 5 minor criteria

Pathological criteria:
Positive histology or microbiology of pathological material obtained at autopsy or cardiac surgery (valve tissue, vegetations, embolic fragments or intracardiac abscess content)

Major criteria:
1) Positive blood cultures
- two positive blood cultures showing typical organisms consistent with infective endocarditis, such as Streptococcus viridans and the HACEK group, or
- persistent bacteraemia from two blood cultures taken > 12 hours apart or three or more positive blood cultures where the pathogen is less specific such as Staph aureus and Staph epidermidis, or
- positive serology for Coxiella burnetii, Bartonella species or Chlamydia psittaci, or
- positive molecular assays for specific gene targets

2) Evidence of endocardial involvement
- positive echocardiogram (oscillating structures, abscess formation, new valvular regurgitation or dehiscence of prosthetic valves), or
- new valvular regurgitation

Minor criteria:
- predisposing heart condition or intravenous drug use
- microbiological evidence does not meet major criteria
- fever > 38 C
- vascular phenomena:
    - ✓ Major emboli,

- splenomegaly;
- clubbing;
- splinter haemorrhages;
- Janeway lesions;
- petechiae or purpura

* immunological phenomena:
    - glomerulonephritis;
    - Osler's nodes;
    - Roth spots

Infective endocarditis prognosis and management:

Poor prognostic factors:
* Staph aureus infection (see below)
* prosthetic valve (especially 'early'; acquired during surgery)
* culture negative endocarditis
* low complement levels

Mortality according to organism:
* staphylococci - 30%
* bowel organisms - 15%
* streptococci - 5%

Current antibiotic guidelines (source: British National Formulary)

Scenario	Suggested antibiotic therapy
Initial blind therapy	Native valve • amoxicillin; consider adding low-dose gentamicin If penicillin allergic, MRSA or severe sepsis: • vancomycin + low-dose gentamicin If prosthetic valve: • vancomycin + rifampicin + low-dose gentamicin
Native valve endocarditis caused by staphylococci	Flucloxacillin: If penicillin allergic or MRSA • vancomycin + rifampicin
Prosthetic valve endocarditis caused by staphylococci	Flucloxacillin + rifampicin + low-dose gentamicin If penicillin allergic or MRSA • vancomycin + rifampicin + low-dose gentamicin
Endocarditis caused by fully-sensitive streptococci (e.g. viridans)	Benzylpenicillin If penicillin allergic: • vancomycin + low-dose gentamicin
Endocarditis caused by less sensitive streptococci	Benzylpenicillin + low-dose gentamicin If penicillin allergic: • vancomycin + low-dose gentamicin

Indications for surgery:

- severe valvular incompetence
- aortic abscess (often indicated by a lengthening PR interval)
- infections resistant to antibiotics/fungal infections
- cardiac failure refractory to standard medical treatment
- recurrent emboli after antibiotic therapy

Infective endocarditis prophylaxis:

The 2008 guidelines from NICE have radically changed the list of procedures for which antibiotic prophylaxis is recommended

NICE recommends the following procedures **do not require prophylaxis:**

- dental procedures
- upper and lower gastrointestinal tract procedures
- genitourinary tract; this includes urological, gynaecological and obstetric procedures and childbirth
- upper and lower respiratory tract; this includes ear, nose and throat procedures and bronchoscopy

The guidelines do however suggest:

- any episodes of infection in people at risk of infective endocarditis should be investigated and treated promptly to reduce the risk of endocarditis developing
- if a person at risk of infective endocarditis is receiving antimicrobial therapy because they are undergoing a gastrointestinal or genitourinary procedure at a site where there is a suspected infection they should be given an antibiotic that covers organisms that cause infective endocarditis

Valvular Ht Disease

Heart sounds

The first heart sound (S1) is caused by closure of the mitral and tricuspid valves whilst the second heart sound (S2) is due to aortic and pulmonary valve closure

S1:

S1 is caused by closure of mitral and tricuspid valves
Causes of a loud S1:
- mitral stenosis
- left to right shunts
- short PR interval, atrial premature beats
- hyperdynamic states

Causes of a quiet or soft S1:
- Long PR
- mitral regurgitation

S2:

- S2 is caused by the closure of the aortic valve (A2) closely followed by that of the pulmonary valve (P2)
- soft in aortic stenosis
- splitting during inspiration is normal

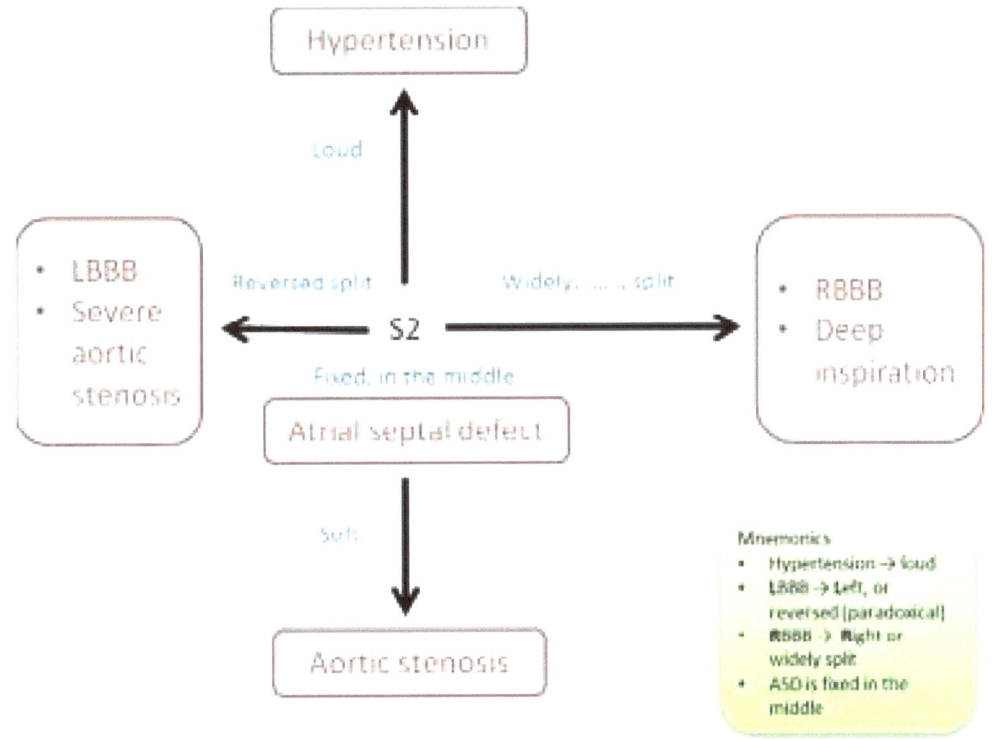

Causes of a loud S2:
- hypertension: systemic (loud A2) or pulmonary (loud P2)
- hyperdynamic states
- atrial septal defect without pulmonary hypertension

Causes of a soft S2:
- aortic stenosis

Causes of fixed split S2:
- atrial septal defect

Causes of a widely split S2:
- deep inspiration
- RBBB
- pulmonary stenosis
- severe mitral regurgitation

Causes of a reversed (paradoxical) split S2 (P2 occurs before A2):
- LBBB
- severe aortic stenosis
- right ventricular pacing
- WPW type B (causes early P2)
- patent ductus arteriosus

S3 (third heart sound)
- caused by diastolic filling of the ventricle
- considered normal if ≤ 30 years old (may persist in women up to 50 years old)
- heard in left ventricular failure (e.g: dilated cardiomyopathy); constrictive pericarditis (called a pericardial knock)

S4 (fourth heart sound):
- may be heard in aortic stenosis, HOCM, hypertension
- caused by atrial contraction against a stiff ventricle
- in HOCM a double apical impulse may be felt as a result of a palpable S4

Mitral stenosis:
- It is said that the 3 causes of mitral stenosis are rheumatic fever, rheumatic fever and rheumatic fever.
- Rarer causes that may be seen in the exam include mucopolysaccharidoses, carcinoid and endocardial fibroelastosis

Features:
- mid-late diastolic murmur (best heard in expiration)
- loud S1, opening snap
- low volume pulse
- malar flush
- atrial fibrillation

Features of severe MS:
- length of murmur increases
- opening snap becomes closer to S2

Echocardiography:
- The normal cross sectional area of the mitral valve is 4-6 sq cm.
- A 'tight' mitral stenosis implies a cross sectional area of ≤ 1 sq cm

Mitral valve prolapse
- Mitral valve prolapse is common, occurring in around 5-10 % of the population.
- It is usually idiopathic but may be associated with a wide variety of cardiovascular disease and other conditions

Associations:
- congenital heart disease: PDA, ASD
- cardiomyopathy
- Turner's syndrome

- Marfan's syndrome, Fragile X
- osteogenesis imperfecta
- pseudoxanthoma elasticum
- Wolff-Parkinson White syndrome
- long-QT syndrome
- Ehlers-Danlos Syndrome
- polycystic kidney disease

Features:
- patients may complain of atypical chest pain or palpitations
- mid-systolic click (occurs later if patient squatting)
- late systolic murmur (longer if patient standing)
- complications: mitral regurgitation, arrhythmias (including long QT), emboli, sudden death

Aortic stenosis

Features of severe aortic stenosis:
- narrow pulse pressure
- slow rising pulse
- delayed ESM
- soft/absent S2
- S4
- thrill
- duration of murmur
- left ventricular hypertrophy or failure

Causes of aortic stenosis:
- degenerative calcification (most common cause in older patients > 65 years)
- bicuspid aortic valve (most common cause in younger patients < 65 years)
- William's syndrome (supravalvular aortic stenosis)
- subvalvular: HOCM
- post-rheumatic disease

Management:
- if asymptomatic then observe the patient is general rule
- if symptomatic then valve replacement
- if asymptomatic but valvular gradient > 50 mmHg and with features such as left ventricular systolic dysfunction then consider surgery
- balloon valvuloplasty is limited to patients with critical aortic stenosis who are not fit for valve replacement

Aortic regurgitation

Features
- early diastolic murmur
- collapsing pulse
- wide pulse pressure
- mid-diastolic Austin-Flint murmur in severe AR - due to partial closure of the anterior mitral valve cusps caused by the regurgitation streams

Causes due to valve disease	Causes due to aortic root disease
- rheumatic fever - infective endocarditis - connective tissue diseases e.g. RA/SLE - bicuspid aortic valve	- aortic dissection - spondylarthropathies (e.g. ankylosing spondylitis) - hypertension - syphilis - Marfan's, Ehler-Danlos syndrome

Bicuspid aortic valve

Overview:
- occurs in 1-2% of the population
- usually asymptomatic in childhood
- the majority eventually develop aortic stenosis or regurgitation
- associated with:
    - ✓ A left dominant coronary circulation (the posterior descending artery arises from the circumflex instead of the right coronary artery) and
    - ✓ Turner's syndrome
- around 5% of patients also have coarctation of the aorta

Complications:
- aortic stenosis/regurgitation as above
- higher risk for aortic dissection and aneurysm formation of the ascending aorta

Tricuspid regurgitation

Signs:
- pan-systolic murmur
- giant V waves in JVP
- pulsatile hepatomegaly
- left parasternal heave

Causes:
- right ventricular dilation
- pulmonary hypertension e.g. COPD
- rheumatic heart disease
- infective endocarditis (especially intravenous drug users)
- Ebstein's anomaly
- carcinoid syndrome

Atrial myxoma

Overview:
- 75% occur in left atrium
- more common in females

Features:
- systemic: dyspnoea, fatigue, weight loss, fever, clubbing
- emboli
- atrial fibrillation
- mid-diastolic murmur, 'tumour plop'
- echo: pedunculated heterogeneous mass typically attached to the fossa ovalis region of the interatrial septum

Murmurs

Ejection systolic:
- aortic stenosis
- pulmonary stenosis, HOCM
- ASD, Fallot's

Holosystolic (pansystolic)
- mitral/tricuspid regurgitation (high-pitched and 'blowing' in character)
- VSD ('harsh' in character)

Late systolic:
- mitral valve prolapse
- coarctation of aorta

Early diastolic:
- aortic regurgitation (high-pitched and 'blowing' in character)
- Graham-Steel murmur (pulmonary regurgitation, again high-pitched and 'blowing' in character)

Mid-late diastolic:
- mitral stenosis ('rumbling' in character)
- Austin-Flint murmur (severe aortic regurgitation, again is 'rumbling' in character)

Continuous machine-like mumur:
- patent ductus arteriosus

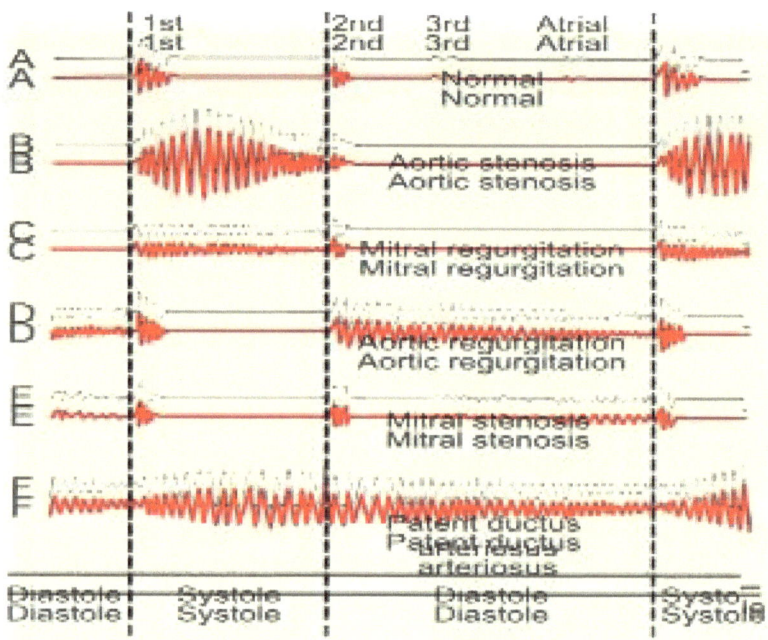

Pulses

Pulsus parodoxus:
- greater than the normal (10 mmHg) fall in systolic blood pressure during inspiration ⇒ faint or absent pulse in inspiration
- severe asthma; cardiac tamponade

Slow-rising/plateau:
- aortic stenosis

Collapsing:
- aortic regurgitation
- patent ductus arteriosus
- hyperkinetic (anaemia; thyrotoxic; fever; exercise/pregnancy)

Pulsus alternans:
- regular alternation of the force of the arterial pulse
- severe LVF

Bisferiens pulse:
- 'double pulse' - two systolic peaks
- mixed aortic valve disease

'Jerky' pulse:
- hypertrophic obstructive cardiomyopathy*

*HOCM may occasionally be associated with a bisferiens pulse

Jugular venous pulse

- As well as providing information on right atrial pressure, the jugular vein waveform may provide clues to underlying valvular disease.
- A non-pulsatile JVP is seen in superior vena caval obstruction.
- Kussmaul's sign describes a paradoxical rise in JVP during inspiration seen in constrictive pericarditis.
- Constrictive pericarditis produces an elevated JVP, with prominent x and y descent

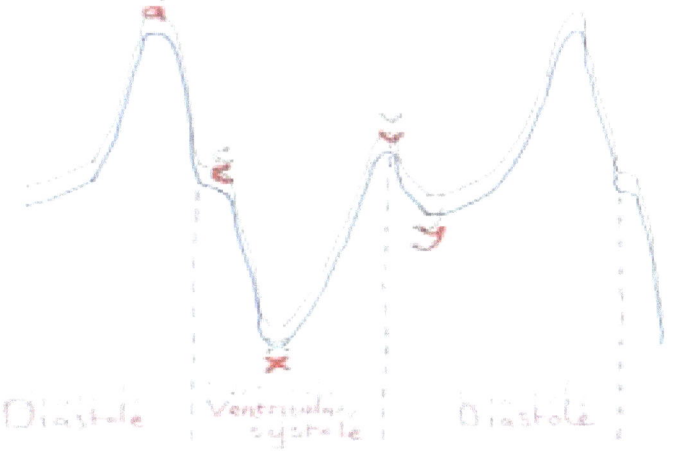

'a' wave = atrial contraction
- large if atrial pressure e.g. tricuspid stenosis, pulmonary stenosis, pulmonary hypertension
- absent if in atrial fibrillation

Cannon 'a' waves:
- caused by atrial contractions against a closed tricuspid valve
- are seen in:
    - Complete heart block,
    - ventricular tachycardia/ectopics,
    - nodal rhythm,
    - single chamber ventricular pacing

'c' wave:
- closure of tricuspid valve
- not normally visible

'v' wave:
- due to passive filling of blood into the atrium against a closed tricuspid valve
- giant v waves in tricuspid regurgitation

'x' descent = fall in atrial pressure during ventricular systole

'y' descent = opening of tricuspid valve

Constrictive pericarditis produces an elevated JVP, with prominent x and y descent

JVP: cannon waves

- Caused by the right atrium contracting against a closed tricuspid valve.
- May be subdivided into regular or intermittent

Regular cannon waves:
- ventricular tachycardia (with 1:1 ventricular-atrial conduction)
- atrio-ventricular nodal re-entry tachycardia (AVNRT)

Irregular cannon waves:
- complete heart block

Prosthetic heart valves

- The most common valves which need replacing are the aortic and mitral valve.
- There are two main options for replacement: biological (bioprosthetic) or mechanical.

Biological (bioprosthetic) valves

- Usually bovine or porcine in origin
- Major disadvantage is structural deterioration and calcification over time.
- Most older patients (> 65 years for aortic valves and > 70 years for mitral valves) receive a bioprosthetic valve
- Long-term anticoagulation not usually needed.
- Warfarin may be given for the first 3 months depending on patient factors.
- Low-dose aspirin is given long-term.

Mechanical valves

- The most common type now implanted is the bileaflet valve.
- Ball-and-cage valves are rarely used nowadays
- Mechanical valves have a low failure rate
- Major disadvantage is the increased risk of thrombosis meaning long-term anticoagulation is needed.
- Aspirin is normally given in addition unless there is a contraindication.

Target INR:
- aortic: 2.0-3.0
- mitral: 2.5-3.5

Following the 2008 NICE guidelines for prophylaxis of endocarditis antibiotics are no longer recommended for common procedures such as dental work.

Congenital Heart Disease

Types:

Acyanotic - most common causes
- ventricular septal defects (VSD) - most common, accounts for 30%
- atrial septal defect (ASD)
- patent ductus arteriosus (PDA)
- coarctation of the aorta
- aortic valve stenosis

VSDs are more common than ASDs. However, in adult patients ASDs are the more common new diagnosis as they generally presents later

Cyanotic - most common causes
- tetralogy of Fallot
- transposition of the great arteries (TGA)
- tricuspid atresia
- pulmonary valve stenosis

Fallot's is more common than TGA. However, at birth TGA is the more common lesion as patients with Fallot's generally presenting at around 1-2 months

Ventricular septal defects

- VSDs are the most common cause of congenital heart disease.
- They close spontaneously in around 50% of cases.
- Congenital VSDs are associated with:
    - ✓ Chromosomal disorders (e.g. Down's syndrome, Edward's syndrome, Patau syndrome) and
    - ✓ Single gene disorders such as ……………
- Non-congenital causes include post myocardial infarction

Features:
- classically a pan-systolic murmur which is louder in smaller defects

Complications:
- aortic regurgitation*
- infective endocarditis
- Eisenmenger's complex
- right heart failure
- pulmonary hypertension: pregnancy is contraindicated in women with pulmonary hypertension as it carries a 30-50% risk of mortality

*aortic regurgitation is due to a poorly supported right coronary cusp resulting in cusp prolapse

Atrial septal defects:

- Atrial septal defects (ASDs) are the most likely congenital heart defect to be found in adulthood.
- They carry a significant mortality, with 50% of patients being dead at 50 years.
- Two types of ASDs are recognised;
    - ostium secundum (the most common)
    - ostium primum

Features:
- ejection systolic murmur;
- fixed splitting of S2
- embolism may pass from venous system to left side of heart causing a stroke

Ostium secundum (70% of ASDs)
- associated with Holt-Oram syndrome (tri-phalangeal thumbs)
- ECG: RBBB with RAD

Ostium primum:
- present earlier than ostium secundum defects
- associated with abnormal AV valves
- ECG: RBBB with LAD; prolonged PR interval

Patent ductus arteriosus

Overview:
- acyanotic congenital heart defect
- connection between the pulmonary trunk and descending aorta
- more common in premature babies, born at high altitude or maternal rubella infection in the first trimester

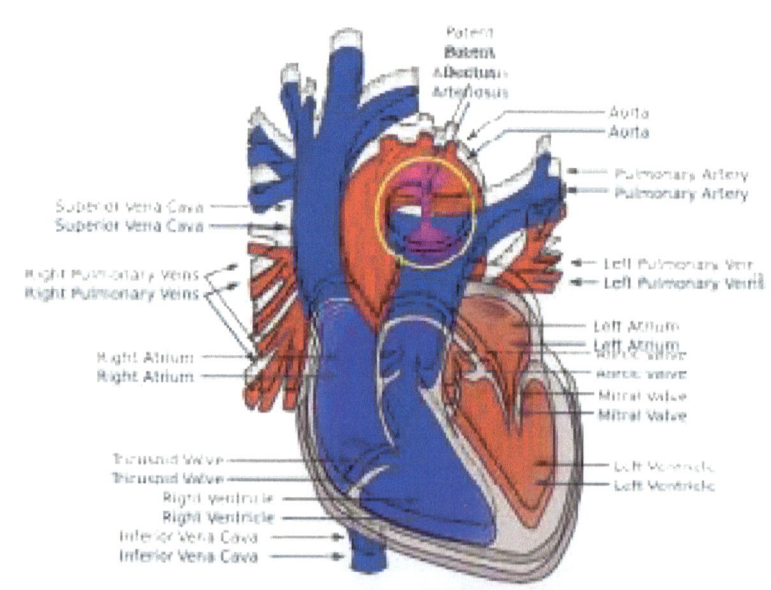

Features:
- left subclavicular thrill
- continuous 'machinery' murmur
- large volume, bounding, collapsing pulse
- wide pulse pressure
- heaving apex beat

Management:
- indomethacin closes the connection in the majority of cases
- if associated with another congenital heart defect amenable to surgery then prostaglandin E1 is useful to keep the duct open until after surgical repair

Patent foramen ovale
- Patent foramen ovale (PFO) is present in around 20% of the population.
- It may allow embolus (e.g. from DVT) to pass from right side of the heart to the left side leading to a stroke - 'a paradoxical embolus'
- There also appears to be an association between migraine and PFO.
- Some studies have reported improvement in migraine symptoms following closure of the PFO

Tetralogy of Fallot
- Tetralogy of Fallot (TOF) is the most common cause of cyanotic congenital heart disease.
- However, at birth transposition of the great arteries is the more common lesion as patients with TOF generally present at around 1-2 months
- It typically presents at around 1-2 months, although may not be picked up until the baby is 6 months old
- TOF is a result of anterior malalignment of the aorticopulmonary septum.
- The four characteristic features are:

    - overriding aorta
    - right ventricular outflow tract obstruction; pulmonary stenosis
    - ventricular septal defect (VSD)
    - right ventricular hypertrophy

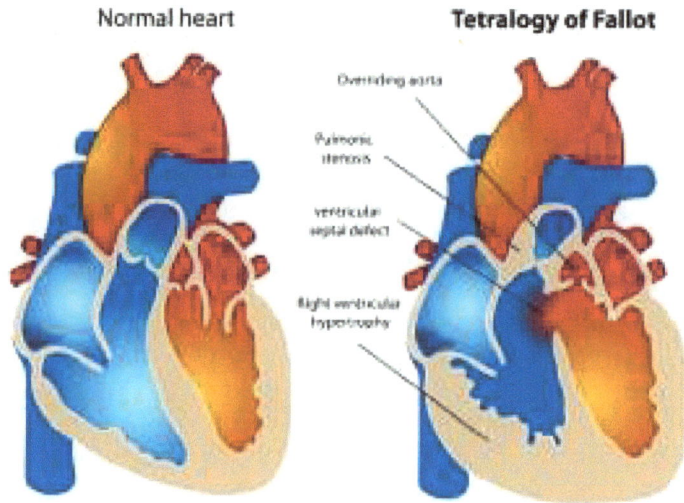

- The severity of the right ventricular outflow tract obstruction determines the degree of cyanosis and clinical severity

Other features:
- cyanosis
- causes a right-to-left shunt
- ejection systolic murmur due to pulmonary stenosis (the VSD doesn't usually cause a murmur)
- a right-sided aortic arch is seen in 25% of patients
- chest x-ray shows a 'boot-shaped' heart, ECG shows right ventricular hypertrophy

Management:
- surgical repair is often undertaken in two parts
- cyanotic episodes may be helped by beta-blockers to reduce infundibular spasm

Eisenmenger's syndrome
- Eisenmenger's syndrome describes the reversal of a left-to-right shunt in a congenital heart defect due to pulmonary hypertension.
- This occurs when an uncorrected left-to-right leads to remodeling of the pulmonary microvasculature, eventually causing obstruction to pulmonary blood and pulmonary hypertension.

Associated with:
- ventricular septal defect
- atrial septal defect
- patent ductus arteriosus

Features:
- original murmur may disappear
- cyanosis
- clubbing
- right ventricular failure
- haemoptysis, embolism

Management:
- heart-lung transplantation is required

Ebstein's anomaly

- Ebstein's anomaly is a congenital heart defect characterised by low insertion of the tricuspid valve resulting in a large atrium and small ventricle.
- It is sometimes referred to as 'atrialisation' of the right ventricle.
- Ebstein's anomaly may be caused by exposure to lithium in-utero

Associations:
- tricuspid incompetence (pan-systolic murmur, giant V waves in JVP)
- Wolff-Parkinson White syndrome

Cardiac imaging:
Non-invasive techniques excluding echocardiography

The ability to image the heart using non-invasive techniques such as MRI, CT and radionuclides has evolved rapidly over recent years.

Nuclear imaging:
These techniques use radiotracers which are extracted by normal myocardium. Examples include:
- thallium
- technetium (99mTc) sestamibi: a coordination complex of the radioisotope technetium-99m with the ligand methoxyisobutyl isonitrile (MIBI), used in 'MIBI' or cardiac Single Photon Emission Computed Tomography (SPECT) scans
- fluorodeoxyglucose (FDG): used in Positron Emission Tomography (PET) scans

- The primary role of SPECT is to assess myocardial perfusion and myocardial viability.
- Two sets of images are usually acquired. First the myocardium at rest followed by images of the myocardium during stress (either exercise or following adenosine / dipyridamole).
- By comparing the rest with stress images any areas of ischaemia can be classified as reversible or fixed (e.g. following a myocardial infarction).
- Cardiac PET is predominately a research tool at the current time

MUGA:
- Multi Gated Acquisition Scan, also known as radionuclide angiography
- radionuclide (technetium-99m) is injected intravenously
- the patient is placed under a gamma camera
- may be performed as a stress test
- Can accurately measure left ventricular ejection fraction.
- **Typically used before and after cardiotoxic drugs are used**

Cardiac Computed Tomography (CT)
- Cardiac CT is useful for assessing suspected ischaemic heart disease;
- uses two main methods:

    1) Calcium score:
        - There is known to be a correlation between the amount of atherosclerotic plaque calcium and the risk of future ischaemic events.
        - Cardiac CT can quantify the amount of calcium producing a 'calcium score'

    2) Contrast enhanced CT: allows visualisation of the coronary artery lumen

- If these two techniques are combined cardiac CT has **a very high negative predictive value** for ischaemic heart disease.

Cardiac MRI:
- Cardiac MRI (commonly termed CMR) has become the gold standard for providing structural images of the heart.
- It is particularly useful when assessing congenital heart disease; determining right and left ventricular mass and differentiating forms of cardiomyopathy.
- Myocardial perfusion can also be assessed following the administration of gadolinium.
- Currently CMR provides limited data on the extent of coronary artery disease.

Please also see the British Heart Foundation link for an excellent summary.

Cardiac catherisation and oxygen saturation levels
- Questions regarding cardiac catherisation and oxygen saturation levels can seem daunting at first but a few simple rules combined with logical deduction can usual produce the answer.
- Let's start with the basics:

    - Deoxygenated blood returns to the right side of the heart via the superior vena cava (SVC) and inferior vena cava (IVC).
    - It has an oxygen saturation level of around 70%.
    - The right atrium (RA), right ventricle (RV) and pulmonary artery (PA) normally have oxygen saturation levels of around 70%

- ✓ The lungs oxygenate the blood to a level of around **98-100%**.
- ✓ The left atrium (LA), left ventricle (LV) and aorta should all therefore have oxygen saturation levels of 98-100%

Some examples:

Diagnosis & notes	RA	RV	PA	LA	LV	Aorta
Normal	70%	70%	70%	100%	100%	100%
Atrial septal defect (ASD)	85%	85%	85%	100%	100%	100%
The oxygenated blood in the LA mixes with the deoxygenated blood in the RA, resulting in intermediate levels of oxygenation from the RA onwards						
Ventricular septal defect (VSD)	70%	85%	85%	100%	100%	100%
The oxygenated blood in the LV mixes with the deoxygenated blood in the RV, resulting in intermediate levels of oxygenation from the RV onwards. The RA blood remains deoxygenated						
Patent ductus arteriosus (PDA)	70%	70%	85%	100%	100%	100%
Remember, a PDA connects the higher pressure aorta with the lower pressure PA. This results in only the PDA having intermediate oxygenation levels						
VSD with Eisenmenger's	70%	70%	70%	100%	85%	85%
PDA with Eisenmenger's	70%	70%	70%	100%	100%	85%
ASD with Eisenmenger's	70%	70%	70%	85%	85%	85%

Angiodysplasia

- Angiodysplasia is a vascular deformity of the gastrointestinal tract which predisposes to bleeding and iron deficiency anaemia.
- There is thought to be an association with aortic stenosis, although this is debated.
- Angiodysplasia is generally seen in elderly patients

Diagnosis:
- colonoscopy
- mesenteric angiography if acutely bleeding

Management:
- endoscopic cautery or argon plasma coagulation
- antifibrinolytics e.g. Tranexamic acid
- oestrogens may also be used

Adult advanced life support

The joint European Resuscitation Council and Resuscitation Council (UK) 2010 guidelines do not alter significantly from the 2005 guidelines. Please see the link for more details, below is only a very brief summary of key points / changes.

Major points include:

- ratio of chest compressions to ventilation is 30:2
- chest compressions are now continued while a defibrillator is charged
- During a VF/VT cardiac arrest, adrenaline 1 mg is given once chest compressions have restarted after the third shock and then every 3-5 minutes (during alternate cycles of CPR).
- In the 2005 guidelines, adrenaline was given just before the third shock. Amiodarone 300 mg is also given after the third shock
- atropine is no longer recommended for routine use in asystole or pulseless electrical activity (PEA).
- a single shock for VF/pulseless VT followed by 2 minutes of CPR, rather than a series of 3 shocks followed by 1 minute of CPR
- asystole/pulseless-electrical activity should be treated with 2 minutes of CPR, rather than 3, prior to reassessment of the rhythm
- delivery of drugs via a tracheal tube is no longer recommended
- following successful resuscitation oxygen should be titrated to achieve saturations of 94-98%. This is to address the potential harm caused by hyperoxaemia

Syncope

Syncope may be defined as a transient loss of consciousness due to global cerebral hypoperfusion with rapid onset, short duration and spontaneous complete recovery. Note how this definition excludes other causes of collapse such as epilepsy.

The European Society of Cardiology published guidelines in 2009 on the investigation and management of syncope. They suggested the following classification:

Reflex syncope (neurally mediated)

- vasovagal: triggered by emotion, pain or stress. Often referred to as 'fainting'
- situational: cough, micturition, gastrointestinal
- carotid sinus syncope

Orthostatic syncope

- primary autonomic failure: Parkinson's disease, Lewy body dementia
- secondary autonomic failure: e.g. Diabetic neuropathy, amyloidosis, uraemia
- drug-induced: diuretics, alcohol, vasodilators
- volume depletion: haemorrhage, diarrhoea

Cardiac syncope

- arrhythmias: bradycardias (sinus node dysfunction, AV conduction disorders) or tachycardias (supraventricular, ventricular)
- structural: valvular, myocardial infarction, hypertrophic obstructive cardiomyopathy
- others: pulmonary embolism

Reflex syncope is the most common cause in all age groups although orthostatic and cardiac causes become progressively more common in older patients.

Evaluation:
- cardiovascular examination
- postural blood pressure readings: a symptomatic fall in systolic BP > 20 mmHg or diastolic BP > 10 mmHg or decrease in systolic BP < 90 mmHg is considered diagnostic
- ECG
- carotid sinus massage
- tilt table test
- 24 hour ECG

DVLA
Cardiovascular disorders
The guidelines below relate to car/motorcycle use unless specifically stated. For obvious reasons, the rules relating to drivers of heavy goods vehicles tend to be much stricter

Specific rules:
-

- Hypertension - can drive unless treatment causes unacceptable side effects, no need to notify DVLA. If Group 2 Entitlement the disqualifies from driving if resting BP consistently 180 mmHg systolic or more and/or 100 mm Hg diastolic or more
- angioplasty (elective) - 1 week off driving
- CABG - 4 weeks off driving
- acute coronary syndrome- 4 weeks off driving; 1 week if successfully treated by angioplasty
- angina - driving must cease if symptoms occur at rest/at the wheel
- pacemaker insertion - 1 week off driving
- Implantable cardioverter-defibrillator (ICD):
    - If implanted for sustained ventricular arrhythmia: cease driving for 6 months.
    - If implanted prophylatically then cease driving for 1 month.
    - Having an ICD results in a permanent bar for Group 2 drivers
- successful catheter ablation for an arrhythmia- 2 days off driving
- Aortic aneurysm of 6cm or more - notify DVLA. Licensing will be permitted subject to annual review.
- An aortic diameter of 6.5 cm or more disqualifies patients from driving
- heart transplant: DVLA do not need to be notified

BY: Ali Ahmed